W9-AVC-194

WITHDRAWN

The 10 Best

Breast Cancer

The Script You Need
to Take Control of Your Health

DEDE BONNER, PH.D.

FOREWORD BY DR. MARISA C. WEISS

A FIRESIDE BOOK
PUBLISHED BY SIMON & SCHUSTER
NEW YORK LONDON TORONTO SYDNEY

DISCLAIMER: This publication contains the opinions and ideas of its author. It is intended to provide helpful and informative material on the subjects addressed in the publication. It is sold with the understanding that the author and publisher are not engaged in rendering medical, health, or any other kind of personal professional services in the book. The reader should consult his or her medical, health, or other competent professional before adopting any of the suggestions in this book or drawing inferences from it.

The author and publisher specifically disclaim all responsibility for any liability, loss or risk, personal or otherwise, which is incurred as a consequence, or directly or indirectly, of the use and application of any of the contents of this book.

NOTE: Dr. Dede Bonner and 10 Best Questions, LLC, own the registered trademarks the 10 Best Questions™, the 10 Worst Questions™, and The Magic Question™.

Fireside
A Division of Simon & Schuster, Inc.
1230 Avenue of the Americas
New York, NY 10020

First Fireside trade paperback edition October 2008

FIRESIDE and colophon are registered trademarks of Simon & Schuster, Inc.

For information about special discounts for bulk purchases, please contact Simon & Schuster Special Sales at 1-800-456-6798 or business@simonandschuster.com.

Designed by Mary Austin Speaker

Manufactured in the United States of America

10   9   8   7   6   5   4   3   2   1

Library of Congress Cataloging-in-Publication Data
    Bonner, Dede.
        The 10 best questions for surviving breast cancer: the script you need to take control of your health / by Dede Bonner.
            p. cm.
        "A Fireside Book."
        1. Breast—Cancer—Popular works. I. Title.
        RC280.B8B63 2008
        616.99'449—dc22   2008006953

ISBN-13: 978-1-4165-6050-0
ISBN-10:   1-4165-6050-5

This book is dedicated to my graduate business stu-

I would like to thank the following people who made this book possible: my devoted husband, Randy Bonner; my loving mother, Jane Anderson; my patient and brilliant editor at Simon & Schuster, Michelle Howry; my literary agent, Paul Fedorko of the Trident Media Group; former Simon & Schuster CEO Jack Romanos; and my attorney, Lisa E. Davis of Frankfurt Kurnit Klein & Selz, PC, all of whom believed in me and in the power of the 10 Best Questions.

I'd also like to thank the experts I interviewed for this book for graciously sharing their time and expertise. Please see their biographies in "Meet the Experts."

Thanks to my university colleagues, Dr. John Fry, Dr. Donald Roberts, and Dr. Ginny Bianco-Mathis of Marymount University in Arlington, Virginia; Dr. Cindy Roman and Dr. Elizabeth B. Davis of the George Washington University in Washington, D.C.; and Dr. Margaret Novak and Dr. Robert Evans of Curtin University of Technology in Perth, Western Australia.

Finally I want to thank my students in the United States and Australia, especially Curtin University student Erika Lozano in Australia and my George Washington University students, Diane Lange Chapman, Jessica Parmalee, and Nichole Peterson, along with their experts on oncology.

by Dr. Marisa C. Weiss

As a newly diagnosed breast cancer patient, a big part of you yearns to close the door on your illness and just pretend this isn't happening to you. You may be worried and anxious about what to expect in the days and weeks ahead. Your emotional roller coaster probably includes feeling helpless, confused, and overwhelmed.

The best way to feel empowered is to know what to expect. You can replace your fears with real information. One key way of getting this information is asking your cancer-care team the questions in this book. Planning and asking questions will help you to rise above your uncomfortable and helpless feelings.

You may be in the habit of taking care of the other people in your life, such as your partner, your children, or your aging parents. Perhaps as a result of being a caregiver, you're less accustomed to the role of needing and receiving care yourself. You may have always looked up to your doctors as being "all-knowing" and powerful, not people to be questioned.

Today there's a great deal more emphasis on a doctor and her patient sharing the decision-making process, as well as many more options for a breast cancer patient to choose from. Sometimes there can be too much information, especially through Internet resources, that it makes knowing what to do or where to turn more difficult and confusing.

That's why asking questions is so valuable. Planning your questions in advance is an empowering technique. It will help you to really stay focused during the short time you have with your doctor during each office visit. Think of planning for your meetings with your cancer-care team as if you were planning for a business meeting. Just as in a business meeting, you want to wear a nice suit, be prepared, and ask smart questions.

A basic premise of asking questions is that it creates a dialogue with your doctors and other medical experts. This dialogue becomes the foundation for establishing a powerful and respectful relationship with your doctors, in which you are actively involved in your own care and treatment.

Patients often worry that their doctors are withholding information, not telling them the whole truth. Sometimes patients think that every word from their doctors is a sign of something important left unsaid. For example, if your surgeon says he'll schedule the lumpectomy within a week, some women automatically jump to the conclusion that this must mean their breast cancer is much worse than their surgeon is telling them, and they're in a state of total panic. A doctor's effort to quickly accommodate your schedule request can make you feel like there's an emergency. This type of misunderstanding is all too common. It often happens because the doctor hasn't communicated well enough with his patient so that she feels she can trust him.

If your doctor understands that you want an active role in your fight against breast cancer, you'll be on the right track to establishing the key elements of a good doctor-patient relationship—trust and respect. A good doctor is one who really listens to your questions and concerns. In my experience, over and over again, this is

time. You should also ask your doctor when she prefers to answer your questions. This helps avoid interruptions and both of you know what to expect.

You want a doctor who will answer your questions. You want to feel that you can really talk with her, that she'll respond directly, carefully, and honestly. From this dialogue and from your "Best Questions" lists, you'll gain more knowledge, reassurance, and the courage to face this disease with an inner strength and fortitude.

Dr. Marisa C. Weiss is the president and founder of the nonprofit organization breastcancer.org, which provides the world's leading online resource for breast health and breast cancer at www.breastcancer.org. She is the co-author with her mother of Living Beyond Breast Cancer, *the author of* 7 Minutes! How to Get the Most from Your Doctor Visit, *and co-author with her teenage daughter of the new book* Taking Care of Your "Girls": A Breast Health Guide for Girls, Teens, and In-Betweens. *Dr. Weiss is also the director of Breast Radiation Oncology and of Breast Health Outreach at Lankenau Hospital in the Philadelphia area.*

The most important questions are often the ones you didn't know to ask. Even the best doctors in the world can't give you the right answers unless you ask them the right questions first.

But how do you know what the right questions are? "Ask your doctor." You've heard it a million times, but do you *really* know what to ask? What if you don't know very much about breast cancer yet, feel intimated by your doctor's expertise, or just feel simply overwhelmed by this diagnosis?

More than ten years ago my mother suffered a major heart attack. As I nervously watched the monitors' readings of her vital signs bounce around, it occurred to me that I didn't know what to ask the doctors about her condition. In that moment of feeling totally helpless, the only thing I could control was my questions. But I just didn't know what to ask.

I vowed to learn how to ask better questions. When I started taking my mom to her follow-up doctor appointments, I spent time researching her medical options and planning questions for her doctor. I wanted to be a well-informed consumer for her sake, to make sure she was getting the very best possible care.

This experience sparked my interest in questioning skills. As I read about questions, I was surprised to learn how little attention people pay to questions in general. It seems that our society is so focused on solutions and answers that we rarely ever stop to consider the quality of our questions.

I started teaching questioning skills as part of the graduate-level business classes I teach in Washington, D.C., and Perth, Australia. My students liked it so much that I developed the concept of "The 10 Best Questions" as a way for them to learn questioning skills, team dynamics, and research skills all at once. For more than five years, I've taught hundreds of students who have interviewed thousands of experts. For example, my students have researched what to ask when you buy a house, get engaged, adopt a dog, hire a financial planner, invest in stocks, retire, plan a wedding, start a diet, and look for great sex.

To learn more about questions, I did a series of interviews with people known for their questioning skills to try to discover their secrets. Helen Thomas, the legendary White House reporter, is famous for her press conference questions to every president since John F. Kennedy. She told me, "Before a news conference I would think, what's the best question to ask? . . . I have the courage of ignorance in my questions. . . . I always get nervous, figuring out what to ask a president. But I believe you have to be curious and keep asking why."

Peter Block, an international management consultant and the author of the book, *The Answer to How Is Yes,* said, "There's a deeper meaning to asking questions. It's a stance you take in the world, a desire to make contact and get connected."

I talked with professional interviewers like Susan Sikora, a TV talk-show host in San Francisco; Debbie Nigro, a New York radio host; and Richard Koonce, a journalist and consultant in Brookline, Massachusetts. From each I heard a version of "you are only as good

waiting to be answered by being asked. Albert Einstein once said, "The difference between me and everyone else is my ability to ask the right questions."

The 10 Best Questions in this book won't make you an instant Einstein. And as "The Question Doctor," I certainly don't claim any Einstein-like brilliance either. I simply believe that a good mind knows the right answers, but a great mind knows the right questions.

Each chapter has a "Best Questions" list, plus one more question that I call "The Magic Question." A "magic question" is the one that even smart people rarely think to ask because it's a "gut-level" question without an obvious answer. I've also tried to include the "best answers" for each question so you'll know when you are hearing the full story.

In writing this book, I've taken a practical and holistic approach to researching the "Best Questions" to make you a "best-informed patient." My focus is to help your decisions, choices, and relationships by suggesting what you can ask your doctors, medical experts, partner, family, friends, and ultimately yourself after a diagnosis of breast cancer.

Your lifetime prescription for good health is to stay informed. Former surgeon general Dr. C. Everett Koop told me he believes, "There's nothing that will lead to better medical care than a knowledgeable patient."

Asking the 10 Best Questions in this book gives you the actual script in hand for each major conversation and decision you will soon be facing in the event of a breast cancer diagnosis. At the same time, be sure to ask plenty of your own questions, too. As Helen Thomas concludes, "There's no such thing as a bad question, only a lot of bad answers."

PART I:

and a fear of failing to communicate well with their doctors. Your medical team can help you make the best decisions, but you have to ask the right questions.

The 10 Best Questions in this section and throughout the book are your action plan, a road map of practical questions and considerations from a holistic point of view for fighting your breast cancer. You don't have to fight this fight alone.

These Best Questions will help to resurrect your sense of control just when you feel the greatest sense of loss and helplessness, help you and your loved ones make sound decisions about choosing top doctors and treatments, and put you firmly in the driver's seat of the "cancer journey" back to good health.

Many people are intimidated by their doctors and are reluctant to ask them questions. Get over it and use this book to help you. Now that you've been diagnosed with breast cancer, a life-threatening disease, this is no time to be shy, to worry about hurting the doctor's feelings or be secretly afraid that he may not like you as much if you ask questions. There's no reason to be aggressive in asking your questions, but be firm in conveying that you expect answers.

To be heard, you may need to repeat your questions or concerns. According to a 1999 study published in *JAMA,* the journal of the American Medical Association, when patients are trying to explain the reason for their visit, doctors typically interrupt after just twenty-three seconds. Persist through interruptions. If your doctor interrupts you before you make your point, try saying, "I'd like to finish" or "Can we come back to my concerns later?"

When you meet with a doctor, have your questions written down and take notes on the answers. You also may want to bring along your partner, a family member, or a close friend to your medical appointments to help you understand and remember.

Many breast cancer specialists and survivors recommend that you also bring a notepad so the person accompanying you can take notes on your behalf; it also helps to bring a tape recorder as well. With a tape recorder, you don't have to worry so much about either of you writing down new medical terms and jargon correctly, and you both can listen more intently and focus on asking questions.

As you are planning your medical appointments, get this book out, review the 10 Best Questions lists, jot down the Best Questions you want to ask, and add your own questions to the list. Take these questions along with you and don't be afraid to ask them.

Let your doctor know at the very beginning of your appointment time that you have questions. Ask the doctor when he or she prefers that you ask your questions. By doing this, you've alerted the doctor to your desire to know more while courteously allowing the doctor to set the pace and timing of the visit.

Just make sure that your questions are answered before time runs out. If not, ask for additional time, another appointment, or whether the doctor will answer your remaining questions by phone or e-mail later.

The Question Doctor wishes you great success and communications with your medical team.

CHAPTER 1: THE 10 BEST QUESTIONS

You, interrupted. That's what a new diagnosis of breast cancer is like. Just as certain as your vivid memories of the day that President John F. Kennedy was shot, the day you watched Space Shuttle *Challenger* and its astronauts dissolve before your eyes, or where you were on September 11, 2001, you will never forget the moment you first learn that you have breast cancer.

Your life changes forever. It seems like the whole universe stops for a moment. Some women describe a sense of slow-motion time, like being in a car accident where it all happens so fast that it seems slow. Things will never be the same.

Beverly Kirkhart, a fifteen-year breast cancer survivor and the co-author of *Chicken Soup for the Surviving Soul: 101 Healing Stories About Those Who Have Survived Cancer*, says that when she first learned she had breast cancer, three things popped into her head. "I had a feeling that I was out of control and had such a sense of loneliness, a feeling of fear that I would lose hope."

Everyone reacts differently. For some women their first reaction after the tears is to learn everything they can about breast cancer. They treat their cancer like a research problem to be solved. Some women call or e-mail every person they have ever talked with since the fifth grade. Others prefer to share the news with only a small circle of family members and friends.

Whatever your initial reaction, whatever moment or stage of

THE QUESTION DOCTOR SAYS:

❯ Don't ever hesitate to ask other questions that are not in this book.

❯ There truly are no dumb questions, especially when you've received a diagnosis of breast cancer. You have every right to know as much as you need to about your cancer.

❯ This is your body and it's your right to have a well-educated mind inside it.

your life has been interrupted by this cancer diagnosis, and no matter who you are, you can benefit from understanding the diagnosis and eventually learning everything you can about breast cancer. You are about to embark on a "cancer journey," a trip you certainly never asked for, but nevertheless the "cancer train" is leaving now with you on it as its unwilling and unprepared passenger. Three decades of studies have all confirmed that a well-educated patient— one who takes charge of her disease and its treatment—has the greatest chance of successfully fighting back cancer and living a normal life.

The following 10 Best Questions are for you to ask when you are first hearing the news that you have breast cancer. This book assumes that you have already had a biopsy and are just now learning its results.

❯❯❯ THE 10 BEST QUESTIONS
About Your Initial Diagnosis of Breast Cancer

1. How sure are you about my diagnosis of breast cancer?

Most women never think to question their diagnosis of breast cancer. If your doctor tells you that you have breast cancer, you probably do.

But breast cancer is complicated and mystifying under a microscope, sometimes even for experienced pathologists, the specialist

THE QUESTION DOCTOR SAYS:

between benign cells (noncancerous) and malignant cells (cancer) is much more complex than you would ever first imagine.

Because of this complexity, the pathology reports diagnosing breast cancer can be wrong. For example, researchers at the Johns Hopkins University in Baltimore, Maryland, found that about 1.4 percent of the time, a pathologist mistakenly diagnoses cancer, misidentifies the type of cancer, or misses a cancer totally. Even more common are pathologists' errors that can significantly change the type of treatment patients receive. These errors can make a world of difference between receiving conservative treatments versus aggressive surgeries.

It's important to make a distinction between raising false hopes for a misdiagnosis and being careful. Your first Best Question when facing breast cancer is to challenge the underlying assumptions that the pathology report is correct. This doesn't mean challenging your doctor's wisdom or credentials, just making sure up front that you aren't jumping on the cancer train when you really don't have a ticket.

Most women will want a second opinion on their diagnosis. See chapter 5 for more explanation on how to do this and the 10 Best Questions to ask for a second opinion.

2. What kind of cancer do I have? What is the medical name?

You will want to name this beast even if the name doesn't mean much to you right now. Ask for the medical name and ask the doctor to write it down for you so you have the correct spelling.

Once you know the medical name and spelling you can look it up on the Internet. Four highly recommended Web sites are those sponsored by the National Cancer Institute (www.cancer.gov), the American Cancer Society (www.cancer.org), breastcancer.org (www.breastcancer.org), and Dr. Susan Love's Web site (www.susanlovemd.com/breastcancer).

3. Where is the tumor located? What size is it?

Knowing where your cancer is located and its size helps make the diagnosis more tangible. Ask your doctor to point out the location of your tumor on the X-ray. Also ask your doctor to draw your tumor's size and shape on a piece of paper for you to take home. Most cancer diagnoses are given in centimeters, which may not make much sense to Americans, who are used to measurements given in inches.

4. How much has the cancer spread? What stage is my cancer and what does that mean in my case?

A critical question about cancer is whether or not it has spread to other organs in your body. Cancer starts when cells begin to divide uncontrollably. Eventually these cells form a visible mass or tumor. This initial tumor is called the **primary tumor.**

Cells from the primary tumor can break off and lodge elsewhere in the body where they then grow into **secondary tumors**. This process is called **metastasis**, which means that the cancer has spread.

Cancer **stages** describe how much the disease has spread. Breast

THE QUESTION DOCTOR SAYS:

cancer has five stages, numbered 0 through IV, with 0 being the earliest stage with the least amount of cancer, and IV being the most advanced cancer stage. If you are told you have a Stage II or III breast cancer, ask if you have Stage IIA, IIB, IIIA, or IIIB, or IIIC for further clarification.

You can also rephrase this question by asking simply if you have a slow-growing breast cancer or an aggressive one. Either way, realize that this is just the start of your education about breast cancer and you'll understand more soon. Cancer staging is important but not necessarily the bottom line of your diagnosis.

5. What is my prognosis? Am I going to die?

This is naturally the first question that jumps to mind for the vast majority of women when they get the initial news about having breast cancer. However, it is purposely Best Question number 5 so you'll learn more about your breast cancer before asking it.

Here's some advice from Betty Rollin, a former NBC correspondent and the author of *First, You Cry*, a groundbreaking book and breast cancer classic that she wrote in 1976 to tell about her breast cancer and mastectomy: "I asked, 'What are my odds?' because I wanted to know the percentages. It was pretty good. It was 80 percent. But I couldn't handle it because that meant I had a 20 percent chance of dying as compared to other people. I asked that question too soon and I regretted it. It's good to be thoughtful about this kind of death question to be sure you can handle the answer before you ask the question. I think it's good to be kind to yourself."

Dr. Betty Ferrell, a veteran of thirty years as an oncology nurse and a research scientist at the City of Hope National Medical Center near Los Angeles, California, says, "All women worry first and foremost about dying."

6. What treatments will I need? When will I start them?

This is another way of saying, "How can I get rid of this awful thing growing inside my breast as fast as possible?"

Many survivors interviewed for this book suggested getting the simplest broad-brush explanation when you first learn about your breast cancer. Chances are, you probably won't hear or understand much anyway at this point—unless you happen to be an oncologist.

An important follow-up question here is, "What happens if I choose to do nothing?" Rather than automatically assuming your best course is to attack this cancer immediately by cutting (surgery), burning (radiation therapy), or poisoning (chemotherapy), ask now what the likely outcomes are if you were to just let it go. You'll never know unless you ask. Choosing to do nothing is one of your options, but it must be a conscious decision reached by you with your doctor, not a denial of your diagnosis, even though it's only natural just to want to turn back the clock and pretend this diagnosis never happened.

7. How long do I have to make decisions about surgery and treatments?

You may be surprised to learn that you have more time than you think before you make decisions and start treatments. Of course, this depends on the type and stage of your cancer and the guidance you receive from your doctor.

...and proactive way of dealing with your disease. Recruit your partner or loved ones as your research assistants so they can be helpful, too.

Most breast cancer cases aren't that urgent, according to many sources such as the National Cancer Institute, the American Cancer Society, and Memorial Sloan-Kettering Cancer Center, a premier cancer facility in New York. You probably have time to learn about your disease and treatment options, as well as find a top oncologist, surgeon, and hospital. In most cases, decisions do not need to be made within a day or two of finding out you have cancer, and taking time to determine the best course of treatment will not affect the outcome of your disease.

Whatever you do, try to put away the terrible burden you feel from a sense of urgency. Confirm the amount of time you have to make a decision with your doctor now, and later with your cancer specialists too.

8. What are the names and contact details of the oncologists and breast surgeons who you recommend to your patients? Why do you recommend these doctors? How well do you know them personally?

Many doctors have a standard list of referrals to local specialists and surgeons, although these doctors may not be breast cancer special-

> *It was such a blow. I was only forty-eight years old. I remember feeling that the floor was caving in on me, that I had been hit with a huge boulder.*
>
> —SUSAN STAMBERG, AWARD-WINNING BROADCAST JOURNALIST FOR NATIONAL PUBLIC RADIO

ists, which is what you should prefer. It's very important to find out why your doctor is referring you to this other doctor and how well these doctors know each other. Then you'll know how reliable this referral really is.

If your doctor gives you several names and not much else, rephrase your question to be, "If your mother had just gotten a diagnosis of breast cancer, which doctor would you send her to first?"

9. Where do you recommend that I be treated? Why do you recommend this hospital or cancer center?

Often the decision about where you get treated will be driven by your choice of oncologist and/or surgeon. Or you can focus your search from the other direction, which is finding a top hospital or cancer center first and then a top doctor at this facility. Be sure to listen to your doctor's reasoning behind his or her referral.

The worst reason is solely because it's a convenient location. You want convenience, of course, but not if you have to sacrifice high quality standards or good success rates with treating breast cancer. You may also be eligible for a clinical trial at a particular center that is somewhat farther away.

10. How can I get more information about my breast cancer? Where can I find emotional, psychological, and spiritual support?

You'll need two kinds of additional information: factual and supportive. Factual information includes objective descriptions of breast cancer types, stages, and treatments. Supportive information will help you meet your emotional, psychological, and spiri-

tual needs as you face down this
diagnosis.

You don't want to bombard the doc-

started. Talk to your doctor about
Web sites, books, and patient education materials to supplement

DR. SUSAN LOVE'S BREAST BOOK,
NOW IN ITS FOURTH EDITION

your knowledge about breast cancer. Also see this book's bibliography and the 10 Best Resources at the end of each chapter.

For supportive information, there are often many community or
Internet resources to help you. These include breast cancer support
groups and trained specialists, such as nurses or oncology social
workers, who are often available for counseling sessions free of
charge at local hospitals or cancer centers.

❯ The Magic Question

What is the most hopeful thing you can tell me about my diagnosis?

Most diagnoses are more hopeful than helpless. Breast cancer is
no longer a death sentence. Millions of women live long, full,
symptom-free, and productive lives after their diagnoses. We can
now detect breast cancer at its earlier, most treatable stage, thanks
to more women receiving routine mammograms and improved diagnostic equipment.

New research and breakthroughs are constantly improving
treatments. Many researchers and cancer experts predict we aren't
far away from making discoveries that will lead to new drugs that

can be targeted precisely and tailored to fit highly individualized treatment plans.

Ask your doctor for your good news. What's the best outcome or longevity you've seen in cases like mine? It will help to put into perspective the bad news about your breast cancer. You deserve some good news today, too.

CONCLUSION

If the first stage of dealing with a diagnosis of breast cancer is shock and emotional distress, the next stage is to learn as much as you can about your options for getting well. The author, the Question Doctor, hopes that you'll find the rest of this book to be a helpful guide and a faithful companion as you take charge of your life again and embark on your brave battle against your breast cancer.

THE 10 BEST RESOURCES

American Cancer Society. "Learn About Breast Cancer." www.cancer.org/docroot/LRN/LRN_0.asp?dt=5.

American Cancer Society. "Talking with Your Doctor: Building a Support Network." www.cancer.org/docroot/ESN/content/ESN_2_2X_Talking_with_your_doctor.asp.

Canadian Cancer Society. "Questions to Ask About Breast Cancer: A Workbook for Women." www.cancer.ca/ccs/internet/standard/0,3182,31 72_236126636_294942259_langId-en,00.html.

Love, Susan, Karen Lindsey, and Marcia Williams. "Part Five: Diagnosis of Breast Cancer and Decisions," in *Dr. Susan Love's Breast Book,* 4th ed. Cambridge: Da Capo Press, 2005.

National Breast Cancer Foundation. "Breast Cancer Library." www .nationalbreastcancer.org/about-breast-cancer/breast-cancer-library.

National Cancer Institute. "What You Need to Know About Breast Cancer." NIH Publication No. 05-1556. www.cancer.gov/cancertopics/wyntk/breast.

PubMed Central. Digital archive of medical and scientific journals. www

Times Books, 1998.

CHAPTER 2: THE 10 BEST QUESTIONS

Most of us believe that our lives might one day depend on the right decision by a doctor, a belief we have about few other professionals. As you face the surprise and suddenness of a diagnosis of breast cancer, that "one day" is no longer abstract. You probably now feel an urgent need to find the right doctor—the one who will help you make the right decisions.

Before you can start getting the cancer care and treatments you need, one of the earliest and potentially scariest decisions you have to make is to find a top oncologist and a top breast surgeon. This may seem like a daunting task unless you happen to have a brother-in-law who is an oncologist or other personal connections.

When describing their worst experiences with doctors, patients often cite arrogance, dismissive attitudes, and "callousness," rather than lack of technical expertise, Ohio State University researchers found in a 2006 study at the Mayo Clinic. So not only do you need a technically capable doctor, but also one with whom you can feel comfortable and who will treat you and your need for knowledge about your disease with respect.

Todd Tuttle, M.D., the chief of surgical oncology at the University of Minnesota, sees the important role of breast surgeons: "The surgeon is usually one of the first breast cancer treatment specialists a woman sees. It's important to choose a surgeon that has good overall understanding of the treatment plan, not just the nuts and bolts of the surgery."

THE QUESTION DOCTOR SAYS:

Be sure to tell your doctor at the beginning of your appointment that you have a list of questions. Ask the doctor when she prefers for you to ask your questions. This way you know her preference for timing and have guaranteed that enough time can be allotted for them. Be politely insistent about getting answers to your questions or have your accompanying loved one ask for you.

Dr. Jerome Groopman in his book *How Doctors Think* says that the best doctors have a relish for knowledge, insatiable curiosity, pride in their performance, and a "clear, clean joy in sharing with you his knowledge" about cancer. Cited among the worst attributes in a doctor are an unwillingness to listen (studies have found that many doctors interrupt patients as often as every twenty-three seconds), a cynical outlook, and the tendency to treat all patients the same (only do one kind of surgery, etc.) with a "cookie cutter" approach to medicine.

The 10 Best Questions in this chapter will help you with the important task of finding a top cancer team—including a medical oncologist who manages cancer treatments, a radiation oncologist who specializes in radiation therapy and a breast surgeon who performs surgery.

〉〉〉THE 10 BEST QUESTIONS
to Find a Top Oncologist or Surgeon

1. Are you board certified? What are your other medical credentials?
Board certification matters.

Board certification assures that the doctor has passed the board requirements for his specialty. In the United States, medical specialty certification is voluntary. Doctors receive their medical licenses after completing medical school and residency requirements.

But this only sets the minimum competency requirements to diag-

maintain board certification, doctors must complete extensive specialty training and pass periodic exams to demonstrate their ongoing competency.

If you are checking on a surgeon, the American College of Surgeons recommends that you look for the following criteria: (1) board certification, (2) hospital or ambulatory center accreditation, and (3) fellowship in the American College of Surgeons. The initials FACS after a doctor's name signifies that he has achieved this fellowship distinction in addition to board certification. Not all surgeons are accepted, while some choose not to become fellows.

State licensure is also very important. Your doctor or surgeon must hold a valid license to practice medicine for the state in which he treats you. Go to the American Medical Association's Web site and click on your state for specific information about a doctor you are considering. Links to state boards can be found at www.ama-assn.org/ama/pub/category/2645.html.

You also want to check on past disciplinary actions and malpractice suits against any doctor or surgeon you are considering. Getting this information is tougher because most doctors and medical associations don't readily disclose unclean histories. Check out ChoiceTrust/HealthPulse, a comprehensive Web site on sanctions and disciplinary actions. This Web site charges a small fee for reports or a one-day pass at www.choicetrust.com. Other sources for checking on prior complaints or disciplinary actions can be found

THE QUESTION DOCTOR SAYS:

If you feel shy or intimidated about asking a potential doctor about credentials, ask his office staff, go to the doctor's Web site or bio, or simply do your own search using this chapter. If you are satisfied about a doctor's credentials, skip asking this question in person. But don't skip this Best Question altogether just because it seems hard to ask. Dig into this doctor's disciplinary history, too. You don't want someone who has served jail time for malpractice holding a scalpel over you!

for free at Docboard.org (www.docboard.org) and Health Care Choices (www.healthcarechoices.org). Additional free services are available from Docinfo (www.docinfo.org) and Consumers' Checkbook (www.checkbook.org).

Also consider where this doctor or surgeon attended medical school, what year he graduated, where he did his residency, how many total years he has been practicing medicine. Often this information is available on a doctor's Web site.

2. What is your experience with my type of breast cancer? How many breast cancer patients did you examine or operate on during the past twelve months?

Experience matters, too. The number of years of total medical practice is significant, along with the years of specialized practice a doctor has in treating breast cancer.

It's very important to determine a doctor's prior experience with your type of breast cancer. One way to determine a doctor's specialized expertise is to ask this follow-up question: "What percentage of your practice is devoted to breast cancer treatment?" The higher the better. You also want to ask, "How many total times have you treated breast cancer?" (for an oncologist) or "How many total breast operations have you done?" (for a surgeon).

If you live in a rural community or have limited access to cancer

will this surgeon be more skillful and confident in the operating room, but she will also be more capable of handling any unforeseen emergencies with your surgery. There's still a lot of truth in Benjamin Franklin's observation, "Beware the young doctor and the old barber." A good rule of thumb is to go with a surgeon who performs this surgery more than just once or twice a year. Ideally, your surgeon specializes in the surgery you need and has additional special training in breast cancer surgery.

A good bedside manner can be very comforting, but don't choose a surgeon based on her personality alone. A surgeon's personality should be the secondary—not the primary—consideration in making your choice. As Shawna C. Willey, M.D., a breast surgeon and the director of the Betty Lou Ourisman Breast Health Center at the Georgetown University Hospital in Washington, D.C., says, "A lot of physicians' skills are judged on their personality. If you have to choose between a good heart and good hands, go with the good hands."

3. May I speak to at least one of your patients to see how they made out in these same circumstances?

This Best Question comes from Dr. C. Everett Koop, the high-profile former U.S. Surgeon General in the 1980s. He believes it's very important to follow through on patient referrals.

Asking for a referral is more common than you might think.

The doctor, surgeon, or the office staff should be ready to offer you at least one name you can call. If not, this may either signal there's something wrong or that the office staff is disorganized. Be sure to follow through with the call, too. Don't procrastinate until it's too late. When you call, it's important to respect the other patient's need for confidentiality.

4. Which hospitals are you affiliated with?

When you need an oncologist or surgeon and a hospital you have two basic choices. You can choose your doctor first and then go with whichever hospital or cancer care center where she has admitting or surgery privileges. This way you are focused on the person and her medical skills.

Or you can choose the hospital or cancer care center first, and then find a top doctor there. In this scenario you are focused first on the facility's expertise or reputation and then the doctor's skills. Many cancer experts stress the importance of going to a comprehensive cancer center if you have this option, but there's no one right approach for every woman with breast cancer. Either way, you want to ask this follow-up question: "What is the accreditation status of this medical facility?"

5. Are you affiliated with any medical schools?

A teaching affiliation with a prestigious medical school is the gold standard when looking for a top oncologist or surgeon. This affiliation is a fairly reliable indicator that this doctor is considered a leader in the cancer field by his peers.

Academic doctors who also practice medicine are likely to be the most well informed about the latest therapies and advances in breast cancer diagnosis and treatment. Not only are they reading medical journals—and writing for them—but they are probably also learning through contacts with their professional colleagues.

most of the jargon or find the articles boring, you can learn a lot about this doctor's interests and approach to treating breast cancer.

Go to PubMed Central (www.pubmedcentral.nih.gov) for a free archive of journal abstracts. Search by the doctor's name. Sometimes the comprehensive cancer center where this doctor works will be cited instead of the individual doctor. Some doctors list their publications with their bios or offer copies to patients as a standard practice.

7. Are you part of a tumor board or a cancer center that holds regular meetings to discuss patients' cases and treatments?

Several doctors interviewed for this book emphasized how important the behind-the-scenes work of a **tumor board** (sometimes called a "tumor team") is for ensuring quality patient care, accurate diagnoses, and effective treatment plans.

This multidisciplinary team typically is composed of cancer experts such as the facility's medical oncologists, radiation oncologists, surgeons, pathologists, mammographers, oncology nurses, and assistants. This team has regular tumor board meetings to discuss the details of recent patient cancer diagnoses and treatment plans. The reason this matters to you is because more heads are better than one in figuring out your breast cancer's "personality," as well as the best course of treatment for fighting it. As J. B. Askew, Jr., M.D., an experienced pathologist in Houston, Texas, explains,

"Pretreatment conferences work by helping everyone who is taking care of a patient to be on the same page . . . This is an extremely powerful way for treatment to begin for a woman with breast cancer."

8. How will you help to involve my family and loved ones in my care decisions? Do you offer support services and more information about breast cancer?

Most women put a lot of value into how attuned a doctor or surgeon is to keeping her partner, family, and other loved ones well informed and involved over time. The doctor's answer to this question will give you a lot of practical information, as well as insights into how patient centered this doctor is. Ideally, you want a doctor who really considers you a whole person and understands that your needs go beyond just physically getting well.

If you have choices, consider going to an oncologist or cancer center that offers support services such as a *nurse navigator* (a specialized nurse with training to help cancer patients) or a trained oncology nurse. As you progress on your cancer journey, you'll have many different needs—including emotional, spiritual, sexual, and healthy lifestyle needs—that can be helped by someone with specialized training. Because it's their job, these specialists are often more readily available, can spend time with you, and may be easier to approach on some highly personal topics, especially with your male doctors.

9. Please describe your preferences for communicating with your patients.

Communication obstacles rank high on most patients' lists of complaints. Communication breakdowns or confusion are additional stressors that you don't need right now with a new diagnosis of breast cancer—and a new doctor.

One of your doctor's roles is to be a good communicator and ex-

cate with you if unanticipated problems come up during your treatment or surgery. Find out if this doctor will take your phone calls or answer e-mails. If so, will you be charged? When's the best time to reach the doctor? In talking with this doctor prior to treatment or surgery, you'll also be able to judge how well the two of you are able to communicate and if you naturally click.

10. Who covers for you when you're on vacation or aren't available?

This is another question that most patients don't think to ask until they can't reach their doctor when they need to. Dr. Willey observes, "It's really the whole experience that matters."

You want to be sure you understand how your doctor can be reached after hours and on weekends, as well as the office's policies and practices concerning partners. For example, you might like your regular doctor but not one of her partners. Sometimes after you arrive for your office appointment, you discover that you'll be seeing the partner instead of your regular doctor. This can be annoying and disruptive, especially with your medical oncologist, whom you'll see for a more extended time than your surgeon or other medical specialists.

"You need to know how to contact your doctor. By knowing how to gain access, it can help you regain a sense of control," says author Dr. Marisa C. Weiss, oncologist and the founder of the popular Web site breastcancer.org.

THREE MORE BEST QUESTIONS FOR SURGEONS

Because a surgeon's skills are uniquely critical to your recovery from breast cancer, here are more Best Questions to ask a prospective surgeon:

1. **If I have excessive pain from my surgery, how will you deal with it?** Melissa Craft, Ph.D., R.N., an advanced oncology nurse in Edmond, Oklahoma, says, "One thing that I've seen is that the surgeons who aren't the best don't have as much concept that things hurt."

2. **How do you do sentinel node biopsies?** The sentinel lymph node is the first lymph node to which cancer is likely to spread from the primary tumor. Cancer cells may appear in the sentinel node before spreading to other lymph nodes. A sentinel lymph node biopsy is a procedure in which the sentinel lymph node is removed and examined under a microscope to determine whether cancer cells are present.

   Breast surgeon Dr. Shawna C. Willey thinks this is an important question that most patients don't know to ask. "Patients should ask what technique is being used because not all sentinel node biopsies are created equal."

3. **For sentinel node biopsies: What is your false negative rate?** Dr. Susan Love explains in *Dr. Susan Love's Breast Book* that a high number of false negatives means the surgeon has repeatedly misidentified the sentinel node. She suggests finding another surgeon if this one balks at this question, is inexperienced with this procedure, or has a high false negative rate.

❯ The Magic Question

What is the most recent thing you learned about breast cancer?

The best answer to this question is not so much what the doctor says but how easily the response rolls off his tongue.

If the doctor is truly an excellent oncologist or surgeon who does enough breast work, he'll be able to tell you something like, "Well, I read an article last week" or "I went to a conference last month." But if the doctor is groping for an answer, that means he doesn't do enough investigation for himself to really know what your best choices for breast cancer care are. Dr. Todd Tuttle com-

practice of medicine, shows evidence of following the new developments, obviously thinks hard about you and your problems, asks questions of you, shows a real interest in your answers, and meets the requirements for board certification and experience, you probably have a good doctor.

Choose a doctor or a surgeon you can trust and feel comfortable with. Many studies have concluded that when a patient is satisfied with her medical care, she is more likely to recover faster and more completely. Use the Best Questions in this chapter as your guide and companion when you're searching for a top doctor.

THE BEST SOURCES FOR FINDING AN ONCOLOGIST OR BREAST SURGEON

It's hard to know where to start when you need an oncologist or surgeon. The following list has been adapted from the National Cancer Institute's list. These sources are either free or have a small fee for use. Spanish language versions are also available.

1. Ask your primary care physician or family doctor. Ask Best Questions 1 and 2 on page 15 and page 17.
2. Ask your family members, friends, coworkers, or breast cancer survivors in support groups.
3. Ask at your local hospital. Some hospitals have patient referral services, but this is likely to be a list of names without recommendations of one doctor over another.
4. National Cancer Institute (NCI) designated Cancer Centers are recognized for their scientific

excellence and extensive resources focused on cancer and cancer-related problems. Start searching at http://cancercenters.cancer.gov.

5. The American Board of Medical Specialties (ABMS) publishes *The Official ABMS Directory of Board Certified Medical Specialists,* which lists doctors' names along with specialties and educational background. See their consumer services at www.abms.org/Who_We_Help/Consumers/. You'll need to register. Or call 866-ASK-ABMS (866-275-2267).

6. The American Medical Association (AMA) DoctorFinder database at http://webapps.ama-assn.org/doctorfinder/home.html provides basic information on licensed physicians in the United States. Users can search for physicians by name or by medical specialty.

7. The American Society of Clinical Oncology (ASCO) provides an online list of doctors who are members of ASCO, more than fifteen thousand oncologists worldwide. It can be searched by doctor's name, institution, location, and type of board certification. Go to www.plwc.org/portal/site/PLWC (click on "Find an Oncologist").

8. The American College of Surgeons (ACS) membership database is an online list of surgeons who are fellows of the ACS. The list can be searched by doctor's name, geographic location, or medical specialty. This service is located at http://web.facs.org/acsdir/default_public.cfm.

9. HealthGrades has a searchable database of doctors. Its reports include doctors' education and training; specialties; board certification; and disciplinary actions. It charges a small fee for reports; www.healthgrades.com.

10. The physician directory at WebMD, a for-profit resource, can help you find doctors' names, contact information, specialties, hospital and HMO affiliations, and driving directions; http://doctor.webmd.com/physician_finder/.

THE 10 BEST RESOURCES

American Board of Medical Specialties. ABMS verification service. www.abms.org.

American Cancer Society. "Worksheet—How to Choose the Right Doctor." www.cancer.org/docroot/ETO/content/ETO_2_2x_how_to_choose_right_doctor_worksheet.pdf.asp.

American Medical Association. "DoctorFinder." www.ama-assn.org/aps/

plinary history. www.docino.org.

Groopman, Jerome. *How Doctors Think.* Boston: Houghton Mifflin, 2007.

HealthGrades. Searchable database of doctors' education, specialties, board certification, and disciplinary actions. www.healthgrades.com.

Love, Susan, Karen Lindsey, and Marcia Williams. "What to Look for in a Doctor and Medical Team," in *Dr. Susan Love's Breast Book,* 4th ed. Cambridge: Da Capo Press, 2005.

National Cancer Institute. "Fact Sheet: How To Find a Doctor or Treatment Facility If You Have Cancer." www.cancer.gov/cancertopics/fact sheet/Therapy/doctor-facility.

U.S. News and World Report. "Best Hospitals 2007 Specialty Search: Cancer." http://health.usnews.com/usnews/health/best-hospitals/search.php? spec=ihqcanc.

You've been told you have breast cancer. Maybe you're feeling overwhelmed, angry, and afraid. One way to move beyond these feelings is to sharpen your mind. It's time to go back to school on one of the most important subjects you'll ever study—learning about breast cancer.

Your diagnosis starts with your pathology report, a description of cells and tissues from your biopsy or surgical tissue sample. A pathology report is written by a pathologist, a medical doctor who specializes in preparing, reviewing, and reporting on tissue samples. Pathologists make a diagnosis of a breast cancer and determine its extent by looking at tissue samples under a microscope.

Understanding your pathology report is critical. It holds the key to your diagnosis, prognosis, and treatment plan. All of your treatment decisions will be based on your pathology report. If your medical oncologist refuses to discuss your pathology report with you or give you a copy of it, find another doctor. You want a doctor who sees teaching you to be a well-informed patient as part of his job.

As advanced oncology nurse Melissa Craft stresses, "I tell my patients, always, always get a copy of your pathology report and have the doctor explain it to you in detail."

This chapter's Best Questions are to be used while your oncologist is reviewing your pathology report with you. It's likely that

THE QUESTION DOCTOR SAYS:

Find out if your oncologist prefers to explain the whole report first and then take your questions or to answer questions on each section. This courtesy will help to build a good relationship with your doctor. Don't be afraid to learn more about your breast cancer. It's what you don't know that can hurt you. You aren't expected by anyone—your doctors, your partner, your loved ones, or yourself—to be a genius about cancer. All you need are the right questions. Let your doctors come up with the right answers.

your doctor will answer these questions without prompting from you. Either way, use these questions to make sure the doctor has discussed the major issues and sections of your pathology report.

SECTIONS OF THE PATHOLOGY REPORT

Here is a brief explanation of the major sections of a pathology report. Each laboratory or cancer center has its own format for its reports. The sections below are based on standardizing guidelines issued by the College of American Pathologists.

1. **Specimen.** Describes where the tissue samples came from, such as from the breast, lymph nodes under your arm, or both.

2. **Clinical history/diagnosis.** Describes the initial diagnosis of breast abnormality prior to the biopsy or surgery.

3. **Gross description.** Describes what the pathologist saw in the tissue samples, including the size, weight, and color of each sample.

4. **Microscopic description.** Describes what the tissues and cancer cells looked like under the microscope.

5. **Special tests or markers.** Describes the results of tests for proteins, genes, and how fast the cells are growing.

first chapter assumed that you were just getting the unpleasant surprise of a diagnosis of breast cancer from a doctor who isn't a cancer specialist, that you wouldn't be fully attentive or emotionally ready for detailed explanations or for medical jargon, and that you didn't have a loved one with you to help you cope and listen better.

Now it's time to ask the doctor to bring on the medical jargon and detailed explanations, preferably while you are holding the hand of someone you love and they are tape-recording this conversation for you.

1. What kind of biopsy did I have? How sure are you of the results?

Your doctor has probably already told you this, but the reason to bring it up again is that some types of biopsies are statistically more likely to be wrong (called **false positives**). The validity of your biopsy sets the stage for deciding if you need a second opinion or another testing procedure to make sure you actually have breast cancer.

There are three main kinds of biopsies:

- **Fine-needle aspiration (FNA).** Just a few cells are taken and analyzed without taking tissue samples. Pathologist Dr. Uthman at Oak Bend Medical Center in Richmond, Texas, explains his reservations about FNA biopsies: "Many pathologists aren't comfortable with FNAs because there are more false positives with them. If your doctor prescribes an FNA for you, really question it because most places [labs] don't want to do them anymore."

- **Core biopsy.** Also called a **needle biopsy.** Similar to a fine-needle aspiration, but your doctor uses a bigger needle to remove the tissue sample for lab evaluation. The drawback to core biopsies, according to Dr. Uthman, is that a small sample may get only the benign changes and miss malignant changes. A reliable and increasingly common procedure in large cancer centers is the use of ultrasound techniques for core biopsies. Another but less frequent practice is the use of the **stereotactic core biopsy.** A stereotactic core biopsy is used when the lesions (abnormal tissue) can only be seen on a mammogram.

- **Surgical biopsy.** Your surgeon removes a tissue sample or lump, typically in outpatient surgery. An **incisional biopsy** takes a sample of a lump or abnormal tissue, while an **excisional biopsy** takes the entire lump or area. When a lump has been discovered but can't be felt and a needle biopsy isn't possible, doctors perform a wire localization procedure in which a thin wire is inserted in the breast before the surgery to provide a cutting guide. This type of biopsy involves anesthesia and a trip to the operating room, so it's becoming a less common practice in large breast care centers, which favor needle biopsies instead.

Don't forget to ask, "How sure are you of the results?" Comprehensive breast care centers are more likely than other facilities to do what pathologist Dr. J. B. Askew calls the "triple test," making sure the results of your biopsy report, the mammographic images (the mammogram and/or ultrasound), and the physical exam all concur. Remember that reading a pathology report is not an exact science. Even the very best pathologist has to take a visual tissue sample and describe it in words. By definition, words and language are subjective and don't have exactly the same

high risk of becoming cancerous), or benign (harmless).

If you are told it's benign, don't just run out the door to celebrate. You still want a copy of the pathology report, because there's one key term you need to look for: **atypical hyperplasia.** If you have this, you have an increased risk of breast cancer in the future. Most pathologists now know how important this is and comment on it in their reports. But don't take any chances. If your report says "hyperplasia of the usual kind," then you're probably fine.

The types of breast cancers are categorized according to how they look under the microscope. Many breast cancers are actually combinations of different types of coexisting cancer cells. It's possible for your biopsy results to come back as one type and a follow-up mastectomy or lumpectomy to show that other types are present in the same tumor. Keep in mind that for now you and your doctor may not know the whole story.

1. **In situ cancers.** Tumors that haven't grown beyond their original site; "in situ" literally means "in the site of," or localized. These are considered noninvasive cancers.

Within in situ cancers there are two types:

A. **Ductal carcinoma in situ (DCIS).** DCIS refers to abnormal cells in the lining of a milk duct that haven't invaded the surrounding breast tissue. This is early stage breast cancer and is sometimes considered a precancerous condition. Almost all women with DCIS can be successfully treated, and no evidence suggests that DCIS affects a woman's life span. However, if left untreated, DCIS may eventually develop into invasive breast cancer.

B. **Lobular carcinoma in situ (LCIS).** LCIS means that abnormal cells are contained within a lobule of your breast but they haven't invaded the surrounding breast tissue. Whether LCIS is an early form of breast cancer or just an indicator for future cancer is still a controversy among experts. But they do agree that LCIS increases the risk of developing breast cancer later on.

2. **Invasive breast cancer.** Also called **infiltrating.** These tumors are capable of growing beyond their original site into the nearby tissue that supports the ducts and lobules of your breast. These cancer cells can travel to other parts of your body, such as the lymph nodes.

There are two types of invasive breast cancer:

A. **Invasive ductal carcinoma (IDC).** IDC accounts for the majority (about 70 percent) of invasive breast cancers. If you have IDC, cancer cells form in the lining of your milk duct, break free from the ductal wall, and invade the surrounding breast tissue. The cancer cells may remain localized—staying near the site of origin—or they can spread **(metastasize)** throughout your body, carried by your bloodstream or lymphatic system.

B. **Invasive lobular carcinoma (ILC).** Although less common than IDC (about 10 percent), this type of breast cancer acts in a similar manner. ILC starts in the milk-producing lobule and invades the surrounding breast tissue. It can also spread throughout your body.

Less common types of breast cancer include the ...

... aggressive), and adenoid cystic carcinoma (invasive but slow growing).

Consult a reputable source, such as the National Cancer Institute or the American Cancer Society, to learn more about your kind of breast cancer, especially if you have a rare type.

3. What is the stage (extent) of my cancer?

Staging is a system that tells you how extensive your cancer is based on established guidelines. It looks at the size of your tumor and whether the cancer has spread to other parts of your body. Your doctor needs this information in order to plan your treatment.

The stage is based on whether the cancer is invasive or not, the size of the tumor, how many lymph nodes are involved, and if the cancer has spread (metastasized) to other parts of your body. Staging a breast tumor can involve a complex calculation and is one of the most important factors in determining your treatment options and prognosis.

Breast cancer has five stages, numbered 0 through IV, with 0 being the least advanced cancer and IV being the most advanced. Here is a brief description of each stage:

Stage 0 is carcinoma in situ. This means it's localized.

Stage I is an early stage of invasive breast cancer. Your tumor is less than 2 centimeters in diameter and cancer cells have not spread beyond the breast.

Stage II   has three scenarios:

IIA.   Your breast tumor is less than 2 centimeters across but the cancer has spread to the lymph nodes under the arm.

IIB.   Your breast tumor is between 2 and 5 centimeters and the cancer may have spread to the lymph nodes under the arm.

IIC.   Your tumor is larger than 5 centimeters (2 inches) but the cancer has not spread to the lymph nodes under the arm.

Stage III   is a locally advanced cancer. The tumor may be large, but the cancer has not spread beyond the breast and nearby lymph nodes. There are three substages with differing degrees of tumor sizes, spread, and advancing complexity.

Stage IV   is metastatic cancer, which means the cancer has spread to other parts of the body.

The TNM Staging System

The most common way to describe the stages of breast cancer is the TNM staging system. It classifies cancers based on their T, N, and M stages:

T   stands for Tumor (its size and how far it has spread within the breast and to nearby organs).

N   stands for spread to lymph Nodes.

M   is for Metastasis (spread to distant organs).

Additional letters or numbers appear after T, N, and M to provide more details about the tumor, lymph nodes, and metastasis. This T, N, and M information is combined in a process called stage grouping. Cancers with similar stages tend to have a similar outlook and thus are often treated in a similar way.

The letter N followed by a number f...

STAGE	T—SIZE OF TUMOR	N—LYMPH NODE STATUS	M—METASTASIS
0	Ductal carcinoma in situ	Negative	None
I	<2 cm	Negative	None
II	0–2 cm	Positive	None
	2–5 cm	Positive or Negative	
III	0–5 cm	Positive (fixed)	None
	>5 cm with skin or chest wall involvement	Positive or Negative (fixed or movable)	
IV	Any size	Any status	Yes

4. What is the size of the tumor at its greatest dimension? Where is it located?

The letter T followed by a number from 0 to 4 describes the tumor's size and spread to the skin or to the chest wall under the breast. Higher T numbers indicate a larger tumor and/or wider spread to tissues near the breast.

Here are all the categories of tumors and their abbreviations:

TX: Primary tumor cannot be assessed.

T0: No evidence of primary tumor.

Tis: Carcinoma in situ (DCIS, LCIS, or Paget's disease of the nipple with no associated tumor mass).

T1 is a tumor between 0 and 2 centimeters.

T2 is a tumor between 2 and 5 centimeters.

T3 is a tumor larger than 5 centimeters.

T4 is a tumor that's growing into the chest wall or skin (includes inflammatory breast cancer).

When you ask about your tumor's location, you'll need a little tumor-site lingo. Think of your breast as if it were a pie marked into four even pieces, called **quadrants.** The four breast quadrants are: (1) upper outer quadrant, (2) lower outer quadrant, (3) upper inner quadrant, and (4) lower inner quadrant. Tumor locations are expressed as straightforward descriptions.

Your treatment plan will be determined in part by the tumor's location. Studies have shown different prognoses and survival rates according to the location of the tumor. For example, a study published in 2007 by the *Annals of Surgical Oncology* concluded that tumor location in the lower inner quadrant is an independent and important prognostic factor for early stage breast cancer. There is growing evidence that tumors of the inner quadrants (especially the lower inner quadrant) metastasize more often.

> *Size matters when it comes to breast cancer, but size is only one of the personality features on the list. You can have a small cancer that behaves like a bully, or a large cancer that is mild mannered.*
>
> —MARISA C. WEISS, M.D., ONCOLOGIST, AUTHOR, AND FOUNDER OF BREASTCANCER.ORG

If you have an inner-quadrant tumor, be sure to ask your d...

...system that

collect and destroy bacteria and viruses. Their white blood cells fight infections and cancer.

Some breast cancers spread to the lymph nodes under a woman's arm. When the lymph nodes are involved in breast cancer, they are called "positive." When lymph nodes are free of cancer, they are called "negative."

Studies show that there's a connection between the number of lymph nodes involved and how aggressive a cancer's personality will be. Usually, the more aggressive cancers have more extensive lymph-node involvement. The total number of lymph nodes involved is more important than the extent of disease within a particular lymph node.

In the TNM staging system, medical experts use the letter N followed by a number from 0 to 3 to indicate whether the cancer has spread to lymph nodes near the breast and, if so, how many lymph nodes are affected.

N0 means no lymph nodes involved.
N1 means 1–3 nodes are involved.
N2 means 4–9 nodes are involved.
N3 means 10 or more nodes are involved.

There are three types of lymph node involvement:

1. **Minimal (or microscopic) lymph node involvement.** Nodes contain only a small number of cancer cells.

2. **Significant (or macroscopic) involvement.** A particular lymph node or group of nodes is cancerous. These nodes can often be felt by hand or seen without a microscope.

3. **Extra-capsular extension.** A tumor takes over a whole lymph node and moves beyond the wall of the lymph node into the surrounding tissue.

Knowing how many of your lymph nodes are affected and the type of lymph node involvement you have will help you and your doctor plan the best treatment regime to fight your cancer.

6. Has the tumor spread, and if so, to what extent?

In the TNM staging system, the M stands for "metastasis," which means the cancer has spread to distant organs, such as your lungs or bones. It is categorized as follows:

MX: Presence of distant spread (metastasis) cannot be assessed.
M0: No distant spread.
M1: Spread to distant organs is present.

7. What are the results of the hormone receptor test?

A hormone receptor test measures the amount of certain proteins, called hormone receptors, in cancer tissue. Hormones can attach to these proteins. A high level of hormone receptors may mean that hormones help the cancer grow.

Hormones such as estrogen and progesterone play a role in the growth of many breast cancers. It is important to know whether a tumor is positive or negative for either of these hormone receptors. An estrogen-receptor-positive tumor is called **ER-positive** (or "ER+") and a progesterone-receptor-positive tumor is called **PR-positive** (or "PR+").

Hormone receptor status is used as a prognostic marker. Hor-

you might benefit from hormone therapy. Hormone therapy is actually therapy with an oral drug, usually tamoxifen or aromatase inhibiters, that blocks hormone receptors in the cancer cell. See chapter 10 for the Best Questions to ask about hormone therapy.

In general, if a patient's cancer is ER positive and PR positive, the patient will have a better-than-average prognosis, and their cancer is likely to respond to hormone therapy (also called "endocrine therapy" or "anti-hormone treatments"). The more receptors present and the more intense their reaction, the more likely the positive response. However, an individual's response depends on a variety of factors. If a patient's cancer is ER negative but PR positive, the patient may still benefit from endocrine therapy but may have a diminished response. If the cancer is both ER negative and PR negative, then the patient will probably not benefit from endocrine therapy.

Hormone receptor status testing is not available in every laboratory. It requires experience and special training to perform and interpret. Your doctor may send your sample to a reference laboratory, and it may take several weeks before your results are available.

8. What are the results of the HER2/neu test? Is it positive or negative?

HER2/neu is a protein that is found on the surface of breast cells. The formal name is "human epidermal growth factor receptor," and it is also known as HER-2, c-erbB-2, ErbB-2, and ERBB2.

The HER2/neu protein sends messages to the cell from growth factors outside the cell. Growth factors tell cells to grow and divide, including cancer cells. The term "overexpression" means there are too many copies of the oncogene (the tumor genes).

Everyone has the HER2/neu protein. But in some breast cancers, the cells produce many more HER2/neu proteins than normal. These breast cancers are called "HER2/neu positive cancers." Breast cancers that have very few HER2/neu proteins, or none at all, are called "HER2/neu negative cancers."

HER2/neu positive breast cancers grow faster than HER2/neu negative breast cancers. This is an important test of your tumor, because it functions not only as a prognostic indictor (HER2/neu positive tumors are more aggressive) but this is also an indicator of the best treatments.

Approximately 25–30 percent of breast cancers have an overexpression (also called "amplification") of the HER2/neu gene. The overexpression of this receptor in breast cancer is associated with increased disease recurrence and worse prognosis. This is not an inherited gene like the ones you get from your mother or father.

Breast cancer scientists and researchers are making progress in finding ways to boost the immune system's ability to fight excess HER2/neu proteins. Treatment drugs are now available, such as Herceptin. Ask your doctor to talk with you about your treatment options if you have an HER2/neu positive breast cancer.

9. Are the margins positive or negative?

The term **margins** means the edges of a tissue sample. The pathology report will tell whether or not there was cancer at the margins of the tissue that was removed. This is a fairly imprecise technique using ink to dye the outside of the tissue sample. The pathologist can only look at representative sections of the margins, so the report on the margins is only an educated guess without 100 ...

... is called **dirty margins**).

Pathologist J. B. Askew, Jr., M.D., explains how to understand margins. "Imagine a hard-boiled egg as the lump removed during a lumpectomy. The yolk is the tumor and the margins are the white part of the egg. We measure what the margins are around every bit of tissue. It's important to know if the whole specimen was processed."

Margin reading is not an exact science and requires a great deal of skill and effort on the part of the pathologist. Pathologists measure the margins to document how closely the in situ and invasive lesions are from each of six margins or edges. Margins are important on mastectomies but are extremely important on lumpectomies, because less tissue is removed.

If there's any doubt in your mind, consider sending your slides to another lab or pathologist for a second opinion. See chapter 5 on getting a second opinion.

10. Please explain my treatment options. Am I a good candidate for participating in a clinical trial?

In this discussion, your oncologist will start to map out her preferences for your care, called a **treatment plan.** When your doctor suggests treatment options, she is taking into account the type of cancer you have, its stage, and how likely these treatment options will work well in your case.

Most women receive chemotherapy, radiation, surgery, or a

combination of the three as part of their breast cancer treatment plan. If your breast cancer is hormone-sensitive (Best Question 7, above), it may be treated with hormone therapy (see chapter 10). Some treatments are experimental and are only available through clinical trials, which are studies used to help researchers understand the safety and efficacy of new treatments.

If you are interested, or even just a little curious, about participating in a clinical trial you need to ask about it now and make a decision fairly quickly. As Dr. Susan Love, best-selling author and breast guru explains, "Most people don't understand that you have to ask [about clinical trials] before your treatments, because if you want to start after the treatment, it's too late! After they've gotten all their treatments, some patients then say, 'I want to be part of a study,' but if it's a study comparing different treatments, you can't do it after the treatment."

❯ The Magic Question

How do you deal with women who have negative biopsies that don't show any cancer, only normal tissue?

If your biopsy had a negative reading, you still want to find out what that means exactly. Pathologist Dr. Edward Uthman explains the importance of this question. "The problem is not so much the positive diagnosis of cancer, but when the biopsy is negative . . . I've learned from experience that some people have to be nagged—it's especially true for a negative biopsy.

"When I get tissue that doesn't have any cancer, there are some pathologists who say, OK, negative biopsy or normal tissue, next case.

"But the first things I want to know are:

- Where did you have this needle?

"If the doctor says, 'Well, if it's negative, I don't worry about it. Get a mammogram in six months.' To me, that would be evidence of someone just going through the motions and not really taking care of his patients. A good doctor would say, 'I don't send patients for biopsies and expect to see negative tissue. I want to talk to that radiologist and find out where he had that needle. I want to talk to the pathologist to find out if what is shown on the slide corresponds to the X-ray. I may even want to get the radiologist and pathologist together to talk it out.' That's someone who goes the extra mile for the patient, not just trying to get through and get to the next patient so he can get his reimbursement."

CONCLUSION

You don't have to face this pathology report alone. Take three things with you. First, take a trusted loved one, someone who is emotionally stable enough to be your listening ears and question asker if you feel a meltdown coming on. Second, take a tape recorder and notepad with you. There will be so much information coming at you that you'll never remember it all. Ask your companion to be in charge of these tasks for you. And third, take these 10 Best Questions as your guide and advisor to make sure your doctor has covered all the important points you need to know. There is nothing more empowering and comforting than to be well informed about your breast cancer and prognosis. Don't be afraid to ask questions or for another explanation of the often frightening and overwhelming pathology report.

THE 10 BEST RESOURCES

American Cancer Society. "Detailed Guide: Breast Cancer." www.cancer.org/docroot/CRI/CRI_2_3x.asp?dt=5.

Askew, J. B., Jr. "What is a Pathology Report?" www.breastpath.com/pathrep.htm.

Breastcancer.org. "Your Pathology Report." www.breastcancer.org/symptoms/path_report/index.jsp.

College of American Pathologists. "Welcome to MyBiopsy.org." www.cap.org/apps/docs/reference/myBiopsy/index2.html.

Elk, Ronit, and Monica Morrow. *Breast Cancer for Dummies*. Hoboken, NJ: Wiley 2003.

Love, Susan, Karen Lindsey, and Marcia Williams. "Pathology Checklist," in *Dr. Susan Love's Breast Book*, 4th ed. Cambridge: Da Capo Press, 2005.

National Cancer Institute. "Pathology Reports: Questions and Answers." www.cancer.gov/cancertopics/factsheet/Detection/pathology-reports.

OncoLink. "Understanding Your Pathology Report: Breast Cancer." www.oncolink.com/types/article.cfm?c=3&s=5&ss=838&id=9588.

Uthman, Edward O., M.D. "The Biopsy Report: A Patient's Guide." cancerguide.org/pathology.html.

Y-ME National Breast Cancer Organization. *Understanding Your Breast Cancer Pathology Report: A Guide for Breast Cancer Patients*. www.y-me.org/publications/generalpubs/read_pathology_report.pdf.

—John Donne,
British poet

Seeing a doctor or a surgeon for the first time is like going on a blind date. You want to find someone you can have a trusted relationship with.

You are probably going on warp speed at this moment, stressed out by your diagnosis. Your head is crammed with a whole new cancer language and reeling with the strange terminology in your pathology report. In other words, you are probably more focused on your disease than your new doctor right now.

Find your favorite quiet spot, draw a soothing bubble bath, or just pull off to the side of the road for a few minutes while you think about your first impressions of the doctor or surgeon you just met with. You'll have time to review your diagnosis and treatment plan, so this may be one of the few times you think hard about your new oncologist or surgeon.

If you have your partner or another loved one with you, both of you can discuss the following Best Questions together. It won't take long, and you shouldn't lose this opportunity.

> *I am appalled, absolutely appalled, at how little doctors say and how many patients come away not having any idea of their case.*
>
> —DR. C. EVERETT KOOP, FORMER U.S. SURGEON GENERAL

>>>THE 10 BEST QUESTIONS
to Assess a Doctor or Surgeon After Your First Consultation

1. How well did the doctor explain my diagnosis? Did he use words that I could easily understand?

The best doctors don't necessarily use the biggest words. What you needed was a simple explanation of your diagnosis and its implications in plain English, not fancy cancer jargon.

Even though this was a dreadful day for you—one you'll never forget—from your doctor's point of view it was routine. Explaining a woman's breast cancer diagnosis is something that breast specialists do all the time. That means that your doctor should have had plenty of opportunities to practice and perfect his spiel before you walked into his office today.

At minimum, your doctor should have showed you your X-rays and given you a copy of your pathology report while explaining the key sections and conclusions. The best doctors are skillful at explaining complex disease processes and treatment plans in simple language. Ideally, your doctor volunteered information that you may not have thought to ask for, such as the possibility of using complementary medicine (see chapter 12) or participating in a clinical trial (see chapter 11), and given you additional sources of information about your type of breast cancer.

2. How well did the doctor listen to me?

Nonjudgmental listening is the key to the most harmonious and effective doctor-patient relationships. An important attribute of a good doctor is that she not only gives answers, but she also asks you questions with a genuine, sincere interest in your answers.

When both parties are listening without bias, they are open to what the other says and thinks. The doctor shouldn't have derided or belittled anything you said or asked.

Good listening skills include these attributes:

- Maintaining eye contact with you
- Not interrupting you
- Leaning toward you while you talked
- Rephrasing what you said for clarity and to check for understanding
- Asking about your feelings and reactions

3. How well did the doctor react to my questions?

Dr. Jerome Groopman, in his bestseller *How Doctors Think,* says, "Patients can help the doctor think by asking questions." The best doctors react positively to questions instead of becoming annoyed, cynical, or angry. They are open to seeing things from your perspective.

If the doctor resented your questions (and you can honestly say that you asked them in a way that was well timed and phrased appropriately), then this negative reaction tells you more about the doctor than about you or your questions. There are no dumb questions. You have every right to ask questions. A doctor's lack of essential communication skills is a deal breaker for most women.

4. What did the doctor's body language tell me about his interest and involvement in my care?

Communication experts tell us that most of us unconsciously read body language when we are talking with others. For example, you can probably tell when your children are getting restless, when your partner is grumpy, or when your mother-in-law wants to go home just by the way they sit, stand, or turn their bodies away from you.

The same happens in doctor-patient relationships. The clues may be subtle, but they are powerful. In fact, those same communication experts say that if we get mixed signals, such as if the doctor is saying nice things but looks bored, we unconsciously believe the body language signal more readily.

Gregory O. Dick, M.D., a reconstructive breast surgeon in Rockville, Maryland, summarizes this Best Question when he says, "You can tell so much by reading the doctor's body language. If the doctor stands away from you in his starched white coat or talks to you with his hand on the door handle on his way out, that tells you so much. You can tell that the doctor is sending the signal that they don't think your questions are important or that they have more important things to do."

5. How comfortable do I feel about working with this doctor?

Comfort level, like trust, is a highly subjective perception. You need a doctor whom you can relax with, have good vibes about, and who treats you with respect. Your doctor should seem interested in you as a person, not just your disease or symptoms.

A doctor's manner is as important as his answers to your questions. Could you confide sensitive information to him? Part of your comfort level comes from your trust in his skills and knowledge. The other part comes from your sense of how nurturing this person

6. How willing is this doctor to be available after regular office hours?

The best oncologists and breast surgeons find ways for you to reach them when you need to, especially in the beginning of your cancer journey, when there are so many unknowns, fears, and decisions to make.

In some large medical practices or cancer centers, doctors share their off-hours duties with partners or have an answering service. Some doctors encourage you to use e-mail or their cell phones after hours. How does this doctor handle his patients after hours? How sincere was he in offering after-hours assistance?

Marti Ann Schwartz, a longtime cancer survivor, patient advocate, and author from Marietta, Georgia, tells her story of finding out the hard way about doctors' office arrangements. "When I was first diagnosed, I saw a doctor who was just sharing the office. I didn't realize the difference, and it was a totally different experience. Make sure the other doctors in the practice are in the same specialty, too."

7. Did the doctor spend enough time with me?

This is a tricky one, because everyone's perception of "enough time" is different. What matters is how you personally feel about the visit. A good doctor doesn't make you feel rushed. She gives you undivided attention.

As Jennifer Armstrong, M.D., a breast cancer medical oncologist with Paoli Hematology Oncology Associates in Paoli, Pennsylvania, comments, "What one patient sees as a negative—for example, feeling rushed in and out—might be seen as a positive by another patient who has a tight schedule and not many questions. Notice how long your wait was, how long other patients were waiting, and compare your wait to how long your visit was. You should feel you had enough time with your doctor."

8. Did this doctor have a problem-solving approach to my cancer treatment that included my family?

Your doctor needs good communication skills to deal with your reactions and questions. Likewise, you want your partner, family, or the loved one who accompanied you to this session to be treated with respect. Positive signs include encouraging and responding well to your loved ones' questions, turning toward them during the conversation, and making frequent eye contact.

Having a problem-solving approach means that your doctor sees you and your loved ones as part of the team that the doctor is assembling to fight your breast cancer. The best doctors know how important your support system and loved ones are to your recovery.

9. What is my impression of the office staff?

Were you and your loved ones greeted warmly? Did you have to wait for a long time to see the doctor? Did the staff seem efficient and courteous? Did they have a copy of your pathology report ready for you when you got there? Did they handle your insurance forms well? Were you offered additional assistance from a nurse, nurse navigator, or access to a social worker?

Or did you feel that you had been dropped into a medical version of a chain eatery, focused on quantity and not the quality of service?

Also think about how well organized your doctor or surgeon

Many of the doctors interviewed for this book and other sources believe that it's a good idea for patients to tape-record their sessions with their doctor, even if they bring a loved one with them to take notes. Some oncologists think that taping is likely to protect them legally as well as help their patients be better informed.

This is especially true when you are reviewing your pathology report with its many confusing new terms and details. Not only can you go back and review the tape later, but there's less pressure on the loved one tasked with taking notes. He is nervous and upset, too, and may miss writing down crucial parts of what the doctor tells you.

The added benefit of tape-recording your medical sessions is that it's another measure of how capable this doctor or surgeon really is. As breast cancer guru Dr. Susan Love says, "You have to worry if the doctor is nervous about having a tape recorder. What's he afraid of? If he's afraid that he's going to get sued by something that he said, then he's not very confident about what he thinks."

❯ The Magic Question

How much did this doctor try to educate me about my breast cancer?

The word "doctor" is from the Latin *docere*, meaning to teach. The medical profession has evolved over time, and now we think of doctoring and teaching as two separate functions.

But the best doctors are still good teachers at heart. Throughout their careers, doctors often find themselves teaching colleagues, other associates, the general public, and their patients.

Rear Admiral Kenneth P. Moritsugu, M.D., former acting U.S. Surgeon General, says, "When the doctor seeks to educate the patient, they are not merely engaging in a two-way conversation. Rather, the doctor is taking it beyond the conversation in order to teach the patient about his or her medical options and how to take control of his or her own health and well-being."

Charles Mayo, cofounder of the legendary Mayo Clinic, once said, "The safest thing for a patient is to be in the hands of a man engaged in teaching medicine." You want your doctor to be your teacher as well as a willing listener. Reflect back on how much time your doctor spent explaining—teaching you—about your disease and treatment options. It's a wonderful indicator of this doctor's most fundamental beliefs about patients as people and as partners—or as just more cancer cases.

CONCLUSION

It's worth it to take the time to assess up front whether or not you feel you have the right doctor or surgeon for you. You are just starting your cancer journey, and you want to ensure that you have every possible advantage on your side.

The ideal doctor is the perfect balance of competence and compassion. He offers both the necessities (skills and experience) and the niceties (easy-going, open) you're looking for.

But keep in mind that no one is perfect, and you may have to make some compromises. These Best Questions, along with the ones in chapters 2, 3, and 5 will help you decide which factors are most important to you in choosing a doctor or surgeon and to what degree a particular doctor or surgeon meets your needs.

By the time you've asked these Best Questions, you'll have really done your homework. Not only will you have found truly the

with_your_doctor.asp.

American Medical Association. "AMA ePhysician Profiles." www.ama-assn.org/ama/pub/category/2672.html.

Boston Central. "Doctor Referrals." www.bostoncentral.com/healthcare/doctor_ref.php.

Cohn, Victor. "How to Recognize the Best Doctors." *Washington Post,* February 2, 1988.

Glazer, James L. "10 Things Patients Need to Hear at Every Visit," *Medical Economics,* November 3, 2006.

Maisano, Gina M. "How to Find a Good Doctor . . . and Recognize a Bad One." *MAMM Magazine,* May–June 2007. www.mamm.com/highlights.php?&qbackid=4667136c872d4f13_34605&qbacktitl=May%20/%20June%202007&seq=2.

Mann, Leslie. "Shopping for a Doctor." *Chicago Tribune,* November 4, 2007.

National Cancer Institute. "Choose Practitioners with Care." www.cancer.gov/cancertopics/thinking-about-CAM/page8.

Reinberg, Steven. "Many Patients Don't Pursue Referrals." www.healthon net.org/News/HSN/606874.html.

U.S. Department of Health and Human Services, Agency for Healthcare Research and Quality. "Quick Tips—When Talking with Your Doctor." www.ahrq.gov/consumer/quicktips/doctalk.htm.

Weiss, Marisa. *7 Minutes! How to Get the Most from Your Doctor Visit.* Philadelphia: Breastcancer.org, 2007.

Seriously consider getting a second opinion after getting a diagnosis of breast cancer. A "second opinion" is defined as seeking another doctor's advice about your diagnosis and treatment. Breast cancer is a very complex and serious disease. According to the Susan G. Komen for the Cure foundation and many other experts, all people who are diagnosed with breast cancer should consider seeking a second opinion. You may also want to seek a second opinion on your pathology report, treatment plan, or almost any aspect of your medical care.

According to several studies over the last ten years, more than one half of all cancer patients get second opinions on their diagnosis or treatments. Women with breast cancer were the most likely of all cancer patients to seek a second opinion. That number is growing as more women become increasingly involved with their own health care and as breast cancer is found at earlier stages, when there are more treatment options.

The good news is that Medicare and most insurance plans will pay for second and even third opinions for cancer. In some cases, insurance plans require second opinions. Check with your health care provider on its specific policies. And though it may take additional time and effort to locate and see another doctor, a delay for this purpose usually won't affect your prognosis. Make sure you discuss with your doctor how much time you have before treatment should begin.

Consider getting your second opinion from one of the National Cancer Institute–designated Cancer Centers around the country or a top cancer hospital. NCI-designated Cancer Centers are recognized for their scientific excellence in treating cancer. See http:// cancercenters.cancer.gov. Chapter 7 has more on cancer hospitals in the United States.

>>>BEST QUESTIONS TO ASK YOURSELF
When Getting a Second Opinion

Use these first five Best Questions to clarify what you want and need in a second opinion before talking with a second doctor.

1. How did I rate my current doctor based on the post-office visit 10 Best Questions assessment list (chapter 4)?

Review your first impressions from those Best Questions and see if any have changed. In addition, this review will help to prepare you mentally for meeting another doctor because you'll be clearer on what matters the most to you.

For example, if you basically liked the first doctor but didn't understand a lot of his explanations, maybe you just ran out of time during your last appointment. Perhaps you were disappointed with the first doctor's staff and realize that you need a more welcoming office environment.

As Dave Balch, founder of the Patient/Partner Project, says about his experiences with his wife, breast cancer survivor Chris, "We didn't feel good about our first doctor. I'm not sure why. He had come highly recommended. We didn't know what to do. I talked with a friend who is an orthopedic surgeon and he said, 'It's really, really important that you feel good about your doctor. Right or wrong, good or bad, if you don't feel...

...whole person?

Unfortunately, study after study suggests that some doctors don't discuss alternative treatments, either because they're too rushed or not knowledgeable themselves. This group includes doctors and surgeons who aren't breast cancer specialists.

Doctors with less experience are not as likely to consider fully the newest breast-conserving surgeries or therapies. This means, for example, that you are more likely to have a mastectomy when only a lumpectomy would have been sufficient. The American Cancer Society makes this point: "There is nothing like a lot of experience when looking for your best treatment."

The other important piece of this assessment is your doctor's interest in you as a person. This is not to suggest that you want to be "bosom buddies" (sorry for the bad pun), but it speaks to how curious this doctor is about you as a unique person. A doctor who is open to learning new things is more likely to be more intelligent, competent, and willing to support you on a personal as well as medical basis.

3. How much do I understand about what I've been told to date about my diagnosis and treatment options?

Think back on your prior sessions with your doctor or surgeon. Look over your notes and listen to tape recordings of your earlier medical appointments.

Confer with your partner or the person who accompanied you to your medical appointments and compare your impressions. Scan this book to learn more about the various types of treatments. All of this will help the factual information to sink in as you step back to assess your situation for a moment.

With this cleared head, try to think through logically how much you truly understand. This is not a reflection of your intelligence, but rather a sign of how well your diagnosis and treatment plan has been explained to you. You want a doctor who is willing and able to put medical jargon into easy-to-understand terms for you and your family.

4. How complicated is my diagnosis and treatment plan?

Don't assume that because you have a straightforward, uncomplicated case of breast cancer that there is nothing to learn and there are no decisions to be made. In most cases, you still have choices.

In studies done by Dartmouth Medical School, researchers found significant treatment differences for cancer surgery and other common procedures among different geographic locations. Doctors' personal beliefs, finances, and medical education are all behind the scenes factors most patients never fully consider. You can't assume that your doctor's recommendation for you is infallible. It is based on his subjective assessment of your case—and even doctors are human and make mistakes. As author, patient advocate, and board-certified surgeon Dr. Vicki Rackner, suggests, "You need a second opinion on everything—the pathology slides, the mammogram, and other imaging studies."

5. What does my inner voice tell me is right for me?

There's a lot to be said for a "woman's instinct" and the value of going with your gut-level reaction. This question suggests that after you've asked all the highly logical, rational, analytical ques-

THE QUESTION DOCTOR SAYS:

tions, you also go with your inner voice, the one that hasn't let you down yet. You need to use both your head and your heart in making your medical decisions.

Malcolm Gladwell, the author of *Blink,* would agree. He says, "We really only trust conscious decision making. But there are moments, particularly in times of stress, when haste does not make waste, when our snap judgments and first impressions can offer a much better means of making sense of the world."

⟩⟩⟩ BEST QUESTIONS TO ASK THE DOCTOR
When Getting a Second Opinion

Use these following Best Questions if you are seeking a second opinion on your diagnosis, pathology report, surgery, treatment plan, or to find another doctor. These are questions to ask the second doctor or medical specialist.

Before you begin searching for a second doctor, get clear what kind of doctor you need and for what specific reason. "Patients need to know what kind of doctor would be most valuable to get a second opinion from. It may be that that doctor is a pathologist, a radiologist, or a surgeon," advises breast surgeon Dr. Shawna C. Willey.

6. How do you interpret my pathology report?

Ask the second doctor to review your pathology report and give you her interpretation of your diagnosis.

There's disagreement among medical experts and breast cancer survivors on whether your second opinion should be "blind." A blind second opinion means that the first doctor's opinion and sometimes the original pathology report and other medical tests aren't shared with the second doctor. The advantage is that the second opinion will be more objective and not influenced by the first one. The drawbacks include putting your second-opinion doctor at a disadvantage by not letting her know the basis for the original diagnosis. A third option is to provide test results, X-rays, and other information without the first doctor's recommendations on diagnosis and treatment.

7. What are the chances that my pathology report could indicate a different diagnosis?

Breast cancer is a complex disease with many factors that need to be considered. One study of breast cancer patients found that the diagnosis changed 20 percent of the time after a second opinion. Breast cancer is expressed in highly individualized ways among patients, and there are few textbook "normal" cases.

A pathology report reading is a subjective interpretation as explained earlier in chapter 3. For example, reading margins (the tissue area surrounding the tumor) is a fairly imprecise technique, especially if the lump is taken out in one piece.

understand what you're being told.

9. Are there any alternative forms of treatment available that my previous doctor may have overlooked? What treatments do you recommend for me?

This question is especially important to ask if your second-opinion doctor is at a large cancer center and has access to the expertise of a multidisciplinary medical team. It just makes sense that more heads are better than one.

There's no need to feel that you are criticizing your first doctor by asking this question. Remember that you are entitled to a second opinion and to be well informed about your choices. You should never have to suffer as a result of a doctor's arrogance or ignorance. If your first doctor does become upset that you want a second opinion, you should choose a different doctor anyway. The best doctors welcome second opinions and even seek them out themselves.

THE QUESTION DOCTOR SAYS:

Reduce the cost and time required for a second opinion by asking your first doctor to send copies of your medical records, X-rays, lab results, and pathology slides/blocks to the second-opinion doctor. And take a loved one and a tape recorder to your session with the second-opinion doctor. That way you'll be able to listen again and later compare your notes on and recordings of the first and second doctors.

10. In your opinion, what is my prognosis? What is my risk of a recurrence of breast cancer after I go through the treatment plan you've outlined for me?

As much as you want to ask this question first, try to refrain until you've given the second doctor a chance to explain how he has interpreted your pathology report and share with you any differences of opinion he has with the first doctor's diagnosis. If you ask about your prognosis too early in the conversation, it'll be very difficult to really listen to much of anything else the doctor says afterward. It's also possible that by listening to the doctor go through his spiel first, before asking this or any other questions, he'll tell you your prognosis during his explanation anyway.

❯ The Magic Question

What advice would you give to your mother (sister, wife) to help her choose between the different recommendations/diagnosis/treatment options I've received?

Getting a second opinion can make things complicated because you may be asked to decide between two different and sometimes even very conflicting opinions. The stakes are high. How can you know which doctor is right?

Rather than try to be the Lone Ranger here and solve this problem yourself, this Magic Question will put the second-opinion doctor's thinking cap on and engage her in helping you make this decision. You can also go back to your first doctor and ask this same question and then compare answers.

Another strategy is to ask the two doctors to confer on your case and see if they can arrive at a mutual opinion. You might also want to ask for a third opinion and then compare all three. Some health insurance providers pay for third opinions for breast cancer patients.

CONCLUSION

...peace of mind about the accuracy of your diagnosis. For all you know (until you ask), your pathologist may not be a breast cancer specialist and you might be a borderline case.

Breast cancer can be a confusing and frightening diagnosis, and it's hard to make decisions about possible treatments. You shouldn't feel rushed or reluctant to get a second opinion because you feel an urgency to take some kind of definitive action to resolve your cancer this very second. Most health insurance providers will pay for a second opinion and some even require it for a diagnosis of breast cancer.

THE 10 BEST RESOURCES

American Cancer Society. "Lack of Information Prompts Search for Second Opinion: Women Want to Know All of Their Options." www.cancer.org/docroot/NWS/content/NWS_1_1x_Lack_of_Information_Prompts_Search_for_Second_Opinion.asp.

American Society of Clinical Oncology. "Find an Oncologist," www.asco.org/ASCO/About+ASCO/Find+an+Oncologist.

Dunn, Steve. "Second Opinions: Why, When, and Who." cancerguide.org/second_opinion.html.

Love, Susan, Karen Lindsey, and Marcia Williams. "Second Opinions," in *Dr. Susan Love's Breast Book*, 4th ed. Cambridge: Da Capo Press, 2005.

National Cancer Institute. "Getting a Second Opinion," in "How to Find a Doctor or Treatment Facility If You Have Cancer." www.cancer.gov/cancertopics/factsheet/Therapy/doctor-facility#second_opinion.

People Living with Cancer. "Seeking a Second Opinion." www.plwc.org/patient/ASCO%20Resources/Find%20an%20Oncologist/Seeking%20a%20Second%20Opinion.

R. A. Bloch Cancer Foundation. "Multidisciplinary Second Opinion Institutions." www.blochcancer.org/articles/xtrnew.asp.

Rosenbaum, Ernest H., Malin Dollinger, and Richard and Annette Bloch. "Cancer Second Opinions." www.cancersupportivecare.com/second_opinions.html.

Yale-New Haven Hospital. "Getting a Good Second Opinion." www.ynhh.org/choice/secondopinion.html.

Y-ME National Breast Cancer Organization. "Breast Cancer Issues for Elderly Women." www.y-me.org/coping/survivorship/survivorship_for_elderly.php.

...... about your health care, but it's hard to know all the facts or where to turn for advice. Most women describe feeling overwhelmed and panicked. Jennie Nash, the author of *The Victoria's Secret Catalog Never Stops Coming, and Others Lessons I Learned from Breast Cancer* and an eight-year breast cancer survivor, recalls her experience: "At a certain point, you realize with some horror that it's *you*! You're the one making the decisions."

There are as many uniquely personal reactions to breast cancer as there are uniquely different manifestations of the disease. Not everyone wants to do a lot of research or become a walking encyclopedia on breast cancer. Others wouldn't have it any other way. Some women reach out to dozens of people for comfort and advice, while others choose to keep their disease private.

Losing a breast is like losing their whole sexual identity for some women, while for others it's less intensely personal. The way women feel about their breasts ranges from women who define their image, appearance, and sexual appeal with their breasts and wearing revealing clothes to other women who barely pay them any mind except in the shower. Some women have little farewell ceremonies before breast surgery, celebrating the feel of the beach's waves, a slinky negligee, or a lover's touch one last time. Other women wish their breast good-bye and good riddance.

Senior researcher and breast specialist Dr. Robert C. Bast, Jr., at the M. D. Anderson Cancer Center in Houston, comments on his observations: "I find an incredible difference in responses to knowing the numbers. Some women will say if there's a 1 percent difference, I'd walk through walls for that. Others say with a 2 or 5 percent difference, do I really want to lose my hair, do I want to feel sick for six months?"

Here's an insider medical perspective on making decisions from author and breast guru Dr. Susan Love: "The truth is that when we give people options it's because there really isn't a best or right answer. So, if we [doctors] think we know the best answer, we don't give options. We say, 'This is what you should do.' But when we say you could do this or you could do that, it's because they really are equal or essentially equal. Therefore there is no best way, and you get to pick which one fits your particular style better."

The 10 Best Questions in this section will help you to strengthen your decision-making muscles. Knowing how you feel, sorting through your personal priorities, and learning about your treatment options will bring you a measure of comfort and self-confidence.

The Question Doctor sincerely hopes the following chapters and Best Questions on treatment choices will ease your cancer journey. Your doctor may be an authority on medicine, but you're the world's foremost expert on yourself.

—Jan King,
author and humorist

Not long ago, the only type of breast cancer surgery was radical mastectomy, which removed the entire breast, along with the chest muscles beneath the breast and all the lymph nodes (glands) under the arm. As breast cancer survivor Jennie Nash observes in her book, *The Victoria's Secret Catalog Never Stops Coming, and Other Lessons I Learned from Breast Cancer,* "This is a good time to get breast cancer. It used to be that a woman got a diagnosis of breast cancer and the next day—no questions asked—she had a mastectomy."

Nowadays, breast cancer patients are usually given surgical choices, and most believe they have every right to ask questions about their surgery. You do. You owe it to yourself to understand as much as possible about your surgery. Literally dozens of research studies all conclude that the best-informed patients recover the quickest because they know what to expect. "Knowing what to expect is an extremely powerful way to minimize your anxiety and the uncertainty," observes oncologist Dr. Marisa C. Weiss.

Most women with breast cancer have some type of breast surgery. This is a decision that you will make along with your oncologist and surgeon, your family, and sometimes with other members of your medical team.

The Best Questions in this chapter will help you to make a

better-educated decision, understand your surgical options, and guide your conversations with your surgeon or oncologist. Having breast surgery is about as much fun as dancing on broken glass, but at least you'll be more ready for it after asking these Best Questions.

>>> THE 10 BEST QUESTIONS
Before Breast Surgery

1. What, if any, viable alternatives to breast surgery do I have? Please describe my nonsurgical options. If none, why do you recommend breast surgery for me?

If you don't ask this question up front, you'll never know if you might have saved yourself the time and discomfort of breast surgery. Since most women with breast cancer, including those with early stages I and II, have some kind of surgery, the chances are that your doctor will recommend surgery for you of some kind.

The follow-up question that might be worth asking, especially if you have very early breast cancer, is, "What happens if I do nothing?" or "What's the least-invasive treatment I can have and still be relatively safe?"

2. Which type of breast surgery do you recommend for me? Why? What are the specific objectives and benefits of this surgery in my case?

You will probably be given the choice between the two main types of breast surgery performed today, breast-conserving surgery and mastectomy. The decision will be based on your diagnosis, your doctors' recommendation, your family history of cancer, and your personal preferences. Knowing your own tolerance for uncertainty will also help you choose between a lumpectomy and mastectomy, and between a mastectomy and a double mastectomy.

gins (edges) of the tissue indicate cancer cells, you may have another surgery known as a **re-excision** to remove more tissue. See more on margins in chapter 3 Best Question 9.

A critical follow-up question when discussing your lumpectomy is to ask the surgeon, "How will the margins be evaluated?" Breast surgeon Dr. Shawna C. Willey explains, "Surgeons discuss this all the time. There's not necessarily a right or wrong answer, but I think you can tell if the surgeon has put some thought into it. Margins have to be marked as the tissue is removed. Marking can be done in several ways, but the main point is that the margins must be oriented."

Following a lumpectomy with radiation therapy is an extra protection against cancer spreading or recurring. See chapter 9 on radiation therapy. If your oncologist also recommends chemotherapy for you after surgery, the radiation therapy may be delayed until chemotherapy is completed. See chapter 8 on chemotherapy.

The second type of breast-conserving surgery is called a **partial** or **segmental mastectomy**. In this surgery, the cancer is removed as well as some of the breast tissue around the tumor and the lining over the chest muscles below the tumor. Usually some of the lymph nodes under the arm are also taken out. Your doctor may recommend the same follow-up treatment plan for radiation therapy and/or chemotherapy following this kind of surgery.

Breast experts generally agree that for most women with early stage breast cancer (I or II), breast-conservation surgery (lumpectomy/partial mastectomy plus radiation therapy) is as effective as mastectomy. The survival rates of women treated with these two approaches are the same.

Mastectomy

During a mastectomy, the surgeon removes the entire breast and sometimes other nearby tissue. There are three main types of mastectomies, simple or total mastectomies, a modified radical mastectomy, and radical mastectomy.

In the first type, called a **simple** or **total mastectomy,** the entire breast is removed but not the underarm lymph nodes or underlying muscles.

In the second type of mastectomy, called a **modified radical mastectomy**, the entire breast and some of the underarm lymph nodes are removed. This is the most common surgery for breast cancer patients who are having the whole breast removed if their sentinel node is involved with the cancer. If you have a smaller tumor, you may be a good candidate for a newer version known as a **skin-sparing mastectomy,** where most of the skin over the breast (other than the nipple and areola) is left intact. If you are considering breast reconstruction surgery, this might be worth talking about with your surgeon.

The third type is a **radical mastectomy.** This is an extensive operation removing the entire breast, axillary (underarm) lymph nodes, and the chest wall muscles under the breast. As noted early, because modified radical mastectomies have been proven to be as effective, radical mastectomies are now rare.

Keep in mind that immediate reconstructive (plastic) surgery is possible for nearly all breast cancer patients. The most important point is choice. Your surgeon should strive to help you understand these surgeries and be a supportive partner in your choice. See more on reconstructive surgery in chapter 13.

Double Mastectomic.

...found that half of the women whom experts deem eligible for lumpectomy chose a mastectomy instead. In fact, an increasing number of women are choosing to have mastectomies over breast-conserving surgery.

Cancer surgeon Todd Tuttle, M.D., has noted a growing number of double mastectomies, especially among younger women. "I think this is an emotional decision. Women want to avoid this awful experience again. But I'm always concerned that this decision is rushed just because of the nature of breast cancer." This trend leads to the next Best Question.

3. How many of each type of breast surgery did you personally perform during the past year? What is your personal preference for performing lumpectomies versus mastectomies?

One of the biggest problems when seeking the advice of a surgeon is trying to understand what his personal biases are. Just like the differences between Republicans and Democrats or liberals and conservatives, everyone has biases, including surgeons.

What in essence you want to understand (and it may be tricky) is how likely your surgeon is to perform one certain breast surgery consistently instead of using the full spectrum of surgical choices. For example, if your surgeon has strong preferences for doing mastectomies, the newest procedures or breast-sparing options might never even be discussed. Older doctors (ones who graduated from medical school before 1981) favor a mastectomy, which was the

THE QUESTION DOCTOR SAYS:

Be sure to ask any other questions you feel are important to understanding your surgery. Don't be intimidated by the surgeon. Surgeons' skills as explainers and listeners vary widely. If you are confused, the surgeon hasn't explained it well enough. Period. It's *not* a reflection of you or your intelligence.

standard breast cancer treatment for years. Mastectomies are less expensive to perform than lumpectomies and pay the doctors more. Poorer women or ones who lack health-care insurance have more mastectomies than women in other socioeconomic groups.

The other factor is fear. Many women are very afraid of a cancer recurrence or radiation therapy, so they choose a double mastectomy even when only one breast has cancer. Double mastectomies are sharply increasing (by 150 percent) between 1998 and 2003, especially among younger women. This trend worries many experts.

It's ultimately your choice about breast surgery if you are a candidate for both lumpectomy and mastectomy. "You don't want a cookie-cutter approach to your surgery," says advanced oncology nurse Melissa Craft. Get a second opinion if you aren't 200 percent convinced that the recommended surgery and surgeon are right for you.

4. Please describe this surgery in simple terms including the exact procedures and how long it will take. Where will this surgery be performed?

Surgeons are required to adhere to the patient-centered principle of informed consent. Although this is often treated as a formality, it's not something to take for granted or lightly. Your surgeon is required to explain the procedure to you and then ask if you fully understand what's going to happen during the surgery. According to the American College of Surgeons, this is ...

... volunteer this information, ask, "Do I need my lymph nodes removed? If so, how many? Why?" Sometimes a few lymph nodes are taken to check for more cancer, a procedure known as **lymph node sampling**, and other times all the lymph nodes under the armpit are removed. This is known as **axillary clearance**.

If your surgeon is planning to remove any or all of your lymph nodes, ask this important follow-up question: "Is a sentinel node biopsy an option in my case?" A **sentinel node biopsy** is a less-invasive way to check for cancer spread in the lymph nodes. Following injections with a tiny amount of radioactive liquid and dye into the area with cancer, the surgeon removes only the sentinel nodes so that they can be tested to see whether they contain cancer cells. The results of research trials suggest that sentinel node biopsy is as effective at detecting cancer cells in the lymph nodes as lymph node sampling or clearance.

Knowing in advance how long the surgery will take will help you judge its extensiveness, as well as let you know how long before your family will be able to see you afterward.

5. What are the short-term and long-term risks for this surgery? Will there be any likely long-term changes from this surgery that won't go away?

Most women are uncomfortable for the first few days after surgery. You are likely to have some postsurgical pain, and obviously your breast will be different. Other possible side effects include infections, hematoma (blood buildup at the wound site), and seroma (fluid buildup). Ask about pain relief before you need it.

For breast-conserving surgery, the most common side effects are pain, temporary swelling, tenderness, and hardness from scar tissue at the surgical site. If your surgeon removes axillary lymph nodes, you may also experience swelling in your arm called **lymphedema.** Lymphedema can be unpleasant and long lasting. Ask your surgeon more about it if lymph nodes are coming out. Some women find that their breast and arm are sore for up to a year or more after the treatment.

Your surgeon's answer should include a thorough explanation of why the benefits of having the recommended surgery outweigh the risks—*in your case*. Don't settle for an abstract discussion or quotes of national statistics. Make sure your surgeon addresses her discussion about risks from the perspective of your body, your breast, and any prior medical conditions you have that could be complicating factors. And don't forget to ask the last piece of this Best Question about permanent side effects.

6. Who will do the actual surgery? Will you have other doctors or medical students who will assist in a major way? Do I have any choice in this matter?

No "bait and switch" allowed in the operating room. You want to know who's holding the knives while you're asleep. Some surgeons have assistants or interns take over portions of their surgeries, especially at teaching hospitals associated with medical schools.

If your surgeon tells you that there will be others operating on you and that you have no voice in the mater, then ask this follow-up question and carefully watch the surgeon's body language and reaction: "Would you allow a member of your family to be operated on

ABOUT ANESTHESIA AND ...

... you lots of questions before surgery to get your medical history.

Here are a few to ask him in return. Are you board certified in anesthesiology? What kind of drugs will I be given and how? What are the risks with this type of anesthesia? If you haven't met your anesthesiologist during a separate, presurgery interview, insist on meeting him or her immediately before your surgery—and before he puts you to sleep!

by this person or persons?" Also request the assistants' medical credentials and experience levels with your type of surgery.

7. What can I expect during my immediate recovery? How long will I be in the hospital? Who will be responsible for my care while I'm in the hospital?

You will be encouraged to get out of bed and start moving around as soon as possible after your surgery. The amount of time you are in the hospital depends on the type of surgery you had. After a lumpectomy or other breast-conserving surgery, you may go home the same day, or at most your hospital stay will be one or two days. Women who have mastectomies or have all their lymph nodes removed stay in the hospital one to three days. If you choose to have reconstructive breast surgery now, especially a flap procedure, this will also increase your time in the hospital.

Make sure you know exactly who will be in charge of your care while you are in the hospital. If your surgeon has partners, will they make the hospital rounds instead of your surgeon? How can you reach your surgeon if you have questions? Who will prescribe pain-killers for you? Get the straight facts on communication channels and procedures now. Otherwise, this can be a source of great frustration and confusion during your hospital stay and later.

8. How long will the healing take? When can I return to work and my daily routines? Exercise? Drive? Will I need someone to help me after I leave the hospital?

Again, your surgeon's answer will vary depending on what type of surgery you are having and other health concerns, such as heart disease or advanced age. Be gentle with yourself. You may feel physically and emotionally exhausted.

Your ability to get back to work and your daily routine will depend on how strenuous your job is and what your daily routines are. For example, if you had a mastectomy and have young children, your surgeon will advise you to avoid lifting or carrying them for a while.

Ask if you will need at-home care, rehabilitation services, or physical therapy as part of your immediate recovery. If so, you'll need to make these arrangements before entering the hospital. Follow your surgeon's advice and schedule for returning to normal activities, including exercise, driving, and sex.

9. What will my breast (or chest) look and feel like after the surgery? Where will the scars be and what will they look like?

All breast surgery leaves some scars. You might find it's actually a relief to discuss how your breast will be different rather than imagining the worst. As cancer surgeon Todd Tuttle, M.D., says, "The best breast surgeons should be experienced in performing skin-sparing mastectomies, know breast reconstruction options, and know how to place surgical incision

...have a mastectomy.

10. What is the most probable outcome from this surgery? How likely is it that this surgery will reduce my risk of recurring or spreading breast cancer?

Dr. Susan Love suggests in the fourth edition of *Dr. Susan Love's Breast Book* "that the 'million dollar question' is, 'Does removing most of the tissue get rid of most of the risk?' " There are no absolute guarantees of zero risk for recurring cancer, even if you have a double mastectomy and the most brilliant surgeon in the world. But your surgeon can tell you about the most probable outcome or the best outcome you can hope for.

❯ The Magic Question

How long has the operating room team worked together?

A good surgeon typically works with the same few anesthesiologists, nurses, and medical assistants. Of course, there are some personnel and shift changes that are unavoidable. But the longer or more frequently a surgical team has worked together—just like any other team—the better they work together. Getting a seasoned surgical team may not be an option for you. It also may not be a deal breaker for choosing a surgeon or hospital. But it's nice if you can get it. And it's probably something that never occurred to you to ask about until now.

THREE MORE QUESTIONS FOR SOME WOMEN

Here are three more Best Questions that most women forget to ask before breast surgery. These may not be critical for you, but you may be glad later that you asked them.

1. Should I donate my own blood prior to surgery as a precaution in case I need a transfusion? (This is an unlikely occurrence, but you may feel some security in knowing you'll get your own blood.)
2. Will my tumor be saved? Where will it be stored and for how long? How can I or future researchers access it later for study or for a clinical trial I might participate in?
3. Should I think about additional surgery at the same time as my mastectomy or lumpectomy, such as breast reconstruction?

CONCLUSION

Be sure to ask any other questions you have besides the ones here. By asking good questions, you'll be making the most of your time with your surgeon and letting her know you will be an active player in this fight against your breast cancer.

THE 10 BEST RESOURCES

American Association of Nurse Anesthetists. "Questions You Should Ask." www.aana.com/ForPatients.aspx?ucNavMenu_TSMenuTargetID=66&ucNavMenu_TSMenuTargetType=4&ucNavMenu_TSMenuID=6&id=136.

American Cancer Society. "Detailed Guide: Surgery for Breast Cancer." www.cancer.org/docroot/CRI/content/CRI_2_4_4X_Surgery_5.asp?sitearea=.

American College of Surgeons. "Patient Education: Partners in Surgical Care." www.facs.org/patienteducation/index.html.

American Society of Anesthesiologists. "Patient Education." www.asahq.org/patienteducation/know.htm.

Love, Susan, Karen Lindsey, ~~~~ ~~~~

National Cancer Institute. "Surgery Choices for Women with Early-Stage Breast Cancer." www.cancer.gov/cancertopics/breast-cancer-surgery-choices.

National Research Center for Women and Families. "Mastectomy v. Lumpectomy: Who Decides?" www.center4research.org/bcancersurgery.pdf.

U.S. Department of Health and Human Services, Agency for Healthcare Research and Quality (AHRQ). "Having Surgery? What You Need to Know: Questions to Ask Your Doctor and Your Surgeon." www.ahrq.gov/consumer/surgery/surgery.pdf.

The prospect of your upcoming surgery is scary enough, even without the prospect of possible hospital infections, adverse drug reactions, and other alarming risks frequently reported in medical journals and the national media.

If your doctor has told you that you need either a lumpectomy or a mastectomy, your next job is to find the very best hospital for your surgery. Yes, this is yet one more decision in the midst of information overload and emotional turmoil. But if you aren't restricted by your choice of doctors or health-insurance coverage, this is a potentially important, and even lifesaving, decision.

You may choose simply to go to the hospital where your doctor has operating privileges. If you have chosen your oncologist and surgeon well and have only a short hospital stay after your surgery, there may be nothing wrong with this choice. Your hospital choices may also be limited by your geographical location or ability to travel to an out-of-town hospital.

However, if you do have hospital choices or want the extra assurance that researching hospitals' quality will give you, the following set of Best Questions for choosing a hospital is a shorthand version of lots of legwork and Internet searches. These questions have been compiled from an analysis of hundreds of questions from more than forty reputable sources, along with an interview

> *Once you have your surgery, that's not the end of the story. You may need significant follow-up care in the hospital itself. You are likely to have an ongoing relationship with this hospital as you go through radiation therapy or chemotherapy. You want to assess up front how responsive the staff will be to your future needs.*
>
> —DR. PAUL SCHYVE, SENIOR VICE PRESIDENT OF THE JOINT COMMISSION

with Dr. Paul Schyve, the senior vice president of The Joint Commission (also known as The Joint Commission on Accreditation of Healthcare Organizations). The Joint Commission is the independent, not-for-profit organization recognized nationwide as the premier organization responsible for assessing and accrediting the quality of 95 percent of all hospital beds in the United States.

〉〉〉THE 10 BEST QUESTIONS
for Choosing a Hospital

1. Does this hospital provide the specialties and services that will best meet my specific needs for my breast cancer surgery?

What matters most to you at this point is this hospital's track record in the specialty of breast cancer surgery. You want a hospital that does lots and lots of breast surgeries, where breast surgeries are performed routinely at least every week, if not every day. There's safety in numbers when it comes to surgeries. Keep in mind that smaller hospitals will naturally have fewer surgeries, so ask for percentages to help you put the numbers into proper perspective.

> *When it comes to choosing a hospital, the bottom line is how many resources does this hospital have for breast cancer?*
>
> —MELISSA CRAFT, R.N. PH.D., ADVANCED ONCOLOGY NURSE

A 2006 study in the *Annals of Surgery* found that a patient's chance of dying during or just after surgery was more closely related to the number of operations the hospital did than the number

to www.tacs.org/cancerprogram/howto.html and clicking on "Find a CoC-Approved Cancer Program Near You."

of operations the surgeon did. In fact, cancer patients who go to hospitals that have more patients with their same type of cancer and surgery needs also have better long-term survival rates.

Paul Schyve, M.D., of The Joint Commission, tells of a New York study of surgeons' performance that surprisingly found that some surgeons' outcomes were well above average in one hospital but the exact same surgeons' outcomes were below average in another hospital. The study shows how important the hospital itself is for successful surgical outcomes.

2. Is this a teaching hospital?

If you have an especially complicated illness or surgery, there may be an advantage in choosing a teaching hospital, according to Dr. Schyve, although just because a facility is not a teaching hospital doesn't mean it lacks quality. In general, teaching hospitals tend to be more current on the latest breast cancer science, medications, and surgical techniques. You may have to balance this advantage with the likelihood of hoards of hovering interns just like the television show *Grey's Anatomy,* taking notes while avoiding eye contact with you.

3. What is this hospital's accreditation status?

There isn't a cut and dried answer to this question, because hospitals' accreditation status can shift up or down over time. Find out if your prospective hospital has a history with conditional accreditations (which require them to make improvements within forty-five days of the inspector's critique) or, even worse, have received a "preliminary denial of accreditation."

The Joint Commission, the top U.S. organization for hospital accreditation, sends its inspectors out for on-site hospital inspections at least every three years. If you drill down on The Joint Commission's Web site (www.jointcommission.org), you can find information on standardized performance measures for surgical care. When checking out a specific hospital, look to see how well this hospital has performed specifically for surgical care. This information is not specific for breast cancer surgeries, and not all hospitals report their surgical data (although most do).

Another reliable source of information is HealthGrades, Inc. (www.healthgrades.com). They offer comprehensive reports on hospital ratings, costs, patient volume, and patient safety for a fee. Their Web site also offers free restaurant-style hospital ratings (one to five stars).

4. Does this hospital appear to be clean?

Cleanliness doesn't guarantee that a hospital has good internal procedures to control infections, but dirty public areas or bathrooms are red flags for potential trouble. Ideally, ask if you can take a short tour of the hospital prior to your surgery. Pay attention to:

- Any odors, including the smell of heavy disinfectants used to mask serious sanitation problems
- Signs of clutter (ancient food trays, messy public areas)

- The physical layout of the ...

... the fact that more people die from hospital-acquired infections than all accidents and homicides combined. If the hospital appears dirty to you, don't go there. Period, end of story.

5. What procedures are in place for patient safety and infection control?

Ask this question even if the hospital looks and smells clean. Statistically, you have a one in twenty chance of getting an infection during your hospital stay, according to a 2007 report by the National Academy of Sciences' Institute of Medicine. About ninety thousand Americans die from a hospital-acquired infection every year. The cost to our national health-care system is an additional billion dollars a year.

Ask if this hospital has an infection consultant or infection control team. These are people responsible for making internal checks for frequent hand washing and the proper disposal of medical waste, such as used needles. Researchers have found that improved infection practices can reduce the rate of in-hospital infection by up to 70 percent.

The good news is that there are things you can do to protect yourself during your hospital stay. Most hospital mistakes are preventable. For example, a consumer group in California cites a study where 45 percent of patients or their families caught medical errors themselves.

You can increase your personal margin of safety while you're in the hospital by asking two simple questions:

- Did you just wash your hands? (for medical and nursing staff)
- What's my name?

Even if it seems silly, ask every medical person who touches you (yes, even your doctor) if he has just washed his hands. It might sound like something your mother would nag about, but this simple question is a proven lifesaver. By asking others who you are, you are helping to ensure that the medical staff is giving the right drug or treatment to the right person. Don't trust the harried hospital staff or overworked doctors to do everything right every time, including hand washing between patients. Being an assertive patient may save your life.

6. Who will have the primary responsibility for my care while I'm in the hospital? Who will communicate with me, my family, and with other members of my medical team?

One of the most common complaints among breast cancer patients during their time in the hospital is that no one seemed to be the central person in charge of their care. This becomes crucial if you need more pain meds, have a drain that needs attention, or are waiting for the release to go home.

Ask this question of both your oncologist and your breast surgeon before checking into the hospital. While you're in the hospital, you may see several new doctors due to the hospital's rotating rounds schedule.

The second part of this question is equally important. You need a clear understanding about what you can expect in terms of communications with your medical team prior to your hospital admittance. Dr. Paul Schwe ... The

... know about them?

It is useful to know your rights as a patient. Every hospital should have a statement of patient rights. You can ask for a copy during hospital admission or before. The statement of patient's rights should cover informed consent, privacy during physical examinations, and the right to refuse participation in hospital research experiments.

When examining the hospital's patient's bill of rights, look for patient-centered phrases, not just statements designed to protect the hospital or doctors from medical malpractice lawsuits. Some hospitals have a patient representative or ombudsman department that you can call about the cold mashed potatoes or rude staff.

8. How conveniently located is this hospital for me and my visitors?

It makes sense that you would prefer the hospital that's most convenient to where you live, especially if you expect your family, children, and friends to visit you. Just knowing you'll be on familiar turf can give you a comforting boost of emotional strength to handle your upcoming surgery and cancer treatments. Being hometown centered can also reaffirm your values, such as the importance of using a religiously affiliated hospital or being treated at the same facility used by your family since your childhood.

You may also need to consider the additional costs associated with child care or transportation. Dave Balch of the Patient/Partner Project has been at his wife Chris's side for five years of out-of-town treatments. He estimates their out-of-pocket costs at more than $46,000, including travel expenses for driving more than 26,000 miles to treatments and appointments, lodging, and restaurant meals.

Ask about the hospital's visiting hours if you expect family and friends to come see you. Look for a hospital with convenient visiting hours and a flexible staff willing to accommodate your requests to let your partner and family stay beyond normal hours or overnight.

But before you pack your slippers and head off to your hometown hospital, consider the key finding of a 2003 study published by the *Journal of the National Cancer Institute*. "Patients who traveled 15 miles or more for their care had one-third the risk of death than those living closer. Moreover, for every 10 miles that a patient traveled for care, the risk of death decreased by 3.2 percent." In other words, the quality of care varies greatly across different regions. One study found wide differences between neighboring towns in the number of recommended surgeries for men with similar cases of prostate cancer. Maybe you can live with a slightly elevated chance at a lower-quality but closer hospital, or maybe you can't. This is your personal decision to be discussed with your doctor and family, and you'll need to take your pocketbook into account.

9. Will my insurance cover the costs at this hospital?

Prior to admittance, you need to check with both the hospital and your health-insurance carrier to determine what percentage of your hospital stay will be paid for. Ask the hospital if they have a written description of their services and fees. You also want to check on available resources if you need financial assistance. Some hospitals provide financial assistance. A hospital-based social worker or oncology nurse navigator can help you with information, resources, and advice.

gist.

In the actual discharge plan, look for nitty-gritty instructions on how to change your bandages and detailed suggestions for sleep and medication schedules after you get home. Make sure that you are given easy-to-understand instructions both orally and then in writing before you check out of the hospital.

Finally, ask what to do if you have questions pertaining to the hospital after you leave, including getting an individual's name and phone number if possible. Once your surgery is over, it's not the end of the story. You are likely to continue with this hospital during your chemotherapy or radiation treatments. A good look at a hospital's discharge procedures can go a long way to helping you assess this particular hospital's overall quality.

❭ The Magic Question

Does this hospital have social workers to assist me? How accessible are they?

Social workers help patients and their families find emotional, social, clinical, physical, and financial support services. The presence of social workers on the hospital staff is a sign of how patient centered a hospital is and what kind of support they will provide during your postsurgical recovery and while you are taking cancer treatments. If a hospital-based social worker is available, ask to meet with her to discuss your needs for support. A good social worker will provide a treasure trove of helpful information and a good listening ear.

CONCLUSION

Using these 10 Best Questions will help you make a more informed hospital choice. Being an informed patient is your best protection against medical errors and infections. Don't let doctors, nurses, or aides brush aside your questions. Overcome your reluctance to speak up. Remain firmly polite as you persevere through your list of questions. Your life or health may depend on it.

THE 10 BEST RESOURCES

American Cancer Society. "How to Choose the Right Hospital." www .cancer.org/docroot/ETO/content/ETO_2_2x_how_to_choose_right_hos pital_worksheet.pdf.asp.

Consumers' Checkbook. "Consumers' Guide to Hospitals." www.check book.org (subscription required).

HealthGrades.com. "Guidelines for Choosing a High-Quality Hospital." www.healthgrades.com.

Inlander, Charles B., and Ed Weiner. *Take This Book to the Hospital with You: A Consumer Guide to Surviving Your Hospital Stay.* Allentown, PA: People's Medical Society, 1997.

Joint Commission, The. "Quality Check." www.jointcommission.org . Accreditation results for specific hospitals.

Leapfrog Group. "Hospital Ratings." www.leapfroggroup.org/cp.

National Cancer Institute. "Cancer Centers List." cancercenters.cancer .gov/cancer_centers/cancer-centers-names.html.

Sherer, David, and Maryann Karinch. *Dr. David Sherer's Hospital Survival Guide: 100+ Ways to Make Your Hospital Stay Safe and Comfortable.* Wash-ington, DC: Claren Books, 2003.

U.S. Department of Health and Human Services

American comedian

Chemotherapy (also called "chemo") is the use of drugs to kill cancer cells. Women who have had their breast cancer surgically removed may be given chemotherapy to destroy any remaining cancer cells elsewhere in the body. Chemotherapy is considered an **adjuvant therapy,** meaning "additional," and is a systemic treatment that involves the whole body. Chemotherapy has clearly proved to improve a woman's chances for being cured of her breast cancer. In cases in which tumors cannot be surgically removed, chemotherapy can help to control the tumors' growth or relieve tumor-related symptoms.

Sometimes chemotherapy is used as the only cancer treatment, but more often it's used along with surgery, radiation therapy, and/ or hormone therapy. When chemotherapy is used to shrink the tumor before surgery or radiation therapy, it's called **neo-adjuvant chemotherapy.**

Chemotherapy affects normal cells as well as cancer cells. The side effects that can result are from chemotherapy's impact on normal cells. The type of side effects that a patient may experience depends on the specific drugs, the dosage, and your tumor's personality, type, and stage. Before you agree to chemotherapy, you want to understand fully why your doctor is recommending it and what the concrete benefits to you will be. Part of that understanding is why

> *We treat a large number of women with chemotherapy to help the ones who will actually benefit from it.*
>
> —ROBERT C. BAST, JR., M.D., VICE PRESIDENT FOR TRANSLATIONAL RESEARCH AT THE M. D. ANDERSON CANCER CENTER.

your doctors think you are a good candidate for chemotherapy. It's important that you have a fully informed and realistic assessment of what exactly chemotherapy can and can't do for you.

Knowing what to expect in advance is one of your best weapons in your fight against breast cancer. The more knowledge you have, the more prepared you will be to collaborate with your medical team to make the best decisions about your cancer treatment. You'll be able to better protect yourself against possible chemotherapy side effects and manage the ones that do occur effectively.

This will not be an easy part of your cancer journey. As Dr. Patricia Ganz, the director of cancer prevention and control research at UCLA's Jonsson Comprehensive Cancer Center in Los Angeles, advises, "Be prepared for the side effects and be knowledgeable. Information is very empowering."

❯❯❯ THE 10 BEST QUESTIONS
About Chemotherapy

1. What is chemotherapy? What is your precise intent for using it? What are the names of the drugs you are proposing for me?

First, you'll need a definition of chemotherapy, which is a cancer treatment with certain chemicals, usually **cytotoxic** (poisonous to cells) drugs. You want to understand the reason you need chemotherapy and your treatment goals from your doctor's perspective.

There are three basic reasons for chemotherapy:

- **Cure the cancer.** D~~~~~~

...~~~~ ~~ ~~~ American Cancer Society, more than one hundred chemotherapy drugs are used in various combinations. Sometimes just one drug is used, but more often chemotherapy works best when it consists of more than one drug. This is called **combination chemotherapy** or a **chemotherapy cocktail.**

Don't let long drug names be intimidating. Ask your doctor to write each one down. Question your doctor on why he has chosen a certain drug or drugs for you. Listen for more explanations about the goals for your chemotherapy in the answer you get back.

An advantage to using more than one drug is that it reduces the chance that you'll become resistant to a particular chemotherapy drug. You and your doctor will decide together which drug or combination of drugs, dosages, delivery method, frequency, and length of treatment are best for you. All of these decisions will depend on your type of cancer, its location, the extent of its growth, how it is affecting your normal body functions, whether you've had chemotherapy before, your general health, and any other health problems, such as heart disease or diabetes.

Also ask your doctor how the drugs will be administered. Chemotherapy is given into your veins through a needle or tiny plastic tube. This is called an IV (intravenous) injection and usually requires that you visit your doctor's office, a hospital, or a clinic for your treatments. Some patients take pills instead of or in addition to IV drugs.

2. What percentage of improvement in my prognosis can I reasonably expect from chemotherapy?

In weighing chemotherapy's risks versus benefits, consider the fact that many breast cancer specialists believe that for women with tumors that are 1 centimeter in diameter or smaller and node negative, the risks from chemotherapy outweigh the benefits. In other words, there are some cases where the toxic side effects of chemotherapy just aren't worth the small percentage of beneficial gain.

As Susan Love, M.D., breast cancer guru and bestselling author, explained during an interview, "You need to find what *really* is the benefit so you can make a decision for yourself. Sometimes 1 or 2 percent is worth it for some people, but most of the time it's not. Your decision needs to be in a context and you need absolute numbers."

If you want to know more, go to the Web site Adjuvant! Online (www.adjuvantonline.com). This is a widely referenced source that helps health professionals and patients with early cancer understand the benefits, risks, and statistical data of different therapies for women like you, of similar age, prior health conditions, and type of cancer. Sign in as a professional and no one will be the wiser (except you). This strategy was recommended by several doctors interviewed for this book.

3. What short-term side effects are possible? How will you help me to manage these side effects?

Chemotherapy affects everyone differently. You may have a lot of side effects, some, or none at all. How you feel will depend on your overall health, the kind of drugs you are getting, and the dosages. But usually chemotherapy makes you feel sick because the drugs are very strong. Chemotherapy drugs are designed to work on quickly dividing

...pain. The most common side effect right after chemotherapy is fatigue, which can range from feeling mildly to extremely tired. Cancer fatigue is different from regular tiredness, and many peo-

for a night out on the town with her. She was so right.

—MICHELLE, THIRTY-EIGHT, COLORADO SPRINGS

ple describe the feeling as being weak, weary, heavy, or slow.

Some women have trouble with vaginal dryness, which can affect sexual pleasure or desire. For premenopausal women, chemotherapy can create chemically induced menopause with associated hormone changes, mood swings, and cessation of periods. More than half of women in this category experience hot flashes during treatments. Recent studies suggest the closer you are in age to natural menopause, the higher the risk for this side effect. See more about premature menopause in chapter 10 on hormone therapy.

Other side effects from chemotherapy include anemia, appetite changes, low platelet counts, constipation, diarrhea, flu-like symptoms, fluid retention, hair loss, infection, infertility, mouth and throat changes, nervous system changes, sexual changes, skin and nail changes, eye changes, and urinary, kidney, and bladder changes. In general, the parts of your body most affected by chemotherapy are the parts that have the fastest-growing cells. These include your skin, hair, and bone marrow; the lining of your mouth, stomach, and intestines; and your blood's red and white cells.

Your doctor's answer to this question should include telling you about the seriousness of any side effects, how long they will last, and her plan to help you manage these side effects. Your doctor should be frank with you about which side effects to expect and what medications or therapies will be able to help you. Infections and anemia are two side effects to ask specifically about.

4. What long-term side effects are possible? How will you help me to manage these side effects? Are there any side effects that may not go away?

Most women's side effects go away after their chemotherapy ends. But sometimes it takes months or even years for all the side effects to go away. It may take a while after your treatment ends for your hair to grow back. Within six weeks you should have some hair growing in, depending on how fast your hair normally grows. Your hair may return with a different color or texture, like black and curly if it was brown and straight before chemotherapy. Also keep in mind that you'll lose not only the hair on your head, but the hair on your arms, legs (that's good news!), pubic hair, and some or all of your other hair, like eyebrows and eyelashes.

You might experience fuzzy thinking, headaches, and sometimes persistent mouth sores, runny eyes and nose, constipation, and diarrhea. There may be blood in your stool or urine, and your gums might stay tender for a while. Chronic fatigue may linger for a while, too, as well as swelling and fluid retention.

Some weight gain is another common side effect of chemotherapy that may linger. The current statistics are that about 50 percent of women gain about ten pounds after treatment ends. Other long-term side effects of chemotherapy include chronic bone marrow suppression and, rarely, second cancers, such as leukemia. Some drugs are more toxic to the heart than others or affect your nerves. But these are rare reactions.

For younger women, a serious long-term consequence of che-

5. What is the chance of each side effect in *my* case?

Because side effects are likely with chemotherapy, it's really important to understand them clearly for you personally, not just for that statistically average woman somewhere out there.

Many doctors are used to talking about side effects from a statistical perspective, like how many patients in past clinical trials experienced hot flashes, poor appetites, or constipation. But you want your doctor to give you his best guess—based on your own medical history and current cancer situation—about what you can expect. This will ease your mind, because you'll have a more realistic picture of what's going to happen.

6. What is my overall treatment plan? How long will each session of chemotherapy take? How long will I be under treatment (number of days or weeks)?

A treatment plan is a little like a casserole. It specifies which drugs (the casserole's ingredients), which dosages (measuring out cups and tablespoons), and the scheduling of treatments (baking time).

Treatment schedules vary widely depending on your type of cancer, how advanced it is, how aggressive it is, the goals of the treatment (curative, control, or easing symptoms), the chemotherapy drugs prescribed for you, how your body reacts to chemotherapy, and your expected and actual side effects. You may receive chemotherapy during a hospital stay, while at home, or in a doctor's office, but most likely you'll be treated on an outpatient basis.

Chemotherapy is given in cycles. A cycle is a period of treatment followed by a rest period. For example, you might receive one week of chemotherapy followed by three weeks of rest. The rest period lets healthy cells rebuild and allows your bone marrow to recover between treatments. Some women have chemotherapy before surgery to shrink the tumor, some women have chemotherapy after surgery to kill off remaining cancer cells, and other women have a combination of surgery, chemotherapy, radiation therapy, and/or hormonal therapy in various orders.

Understanding your total time commitment and total treatment plan early on will help you plan your daily life over those next few weeks. While you're undergoing treatment, you may need to work out arrangements for getting rides to your appointments, taking time off from work, and for child care. It'll be easier to plan your personal life if you know in advance how your chemotherapy fits into the total treatment plan that your medical team is suggesting for you.

7. How will my daily life be affected during and after treatments? Will I need someone to take care of me?

Many women are able to continue working or carry on with their usual daily routines while they are undergoing chemotherapy, just as long as they match their schedule to how they feel. While some women find they are able to lead a fairly normal life during their treatment, others become very tired and have to take things much more slowly.

You'll probably want to know as much as possible in advance if you'll be too tired to work full time, care for your children, or keep up with your other normal responsibilities. You may get to a point during your chemotherapy when you feel too sick to work. Talk

8. What, if any, restrictions will there be on my normal activities while I'm undergoing treatment?

This question covers exercise, diet, sex, smoking, drinking alcohol, taking herbs or supplements, driving, working, and special concerns if you are pregnant. Be sure to tell your doctor if you are using complementary medicine, which could affect the chemotherapy's effects. See chapter 12 on complementary medicine.

9. What symptoms or changes in my body are serious enough to warrant my calling you?

This is an important Best Question so you won't worry needlessly or hesitate to take action when you should. Rather than trying to figure out when to call your doctor, let him give you guidelines.

In general, medical experts advise that you need to pay attention to:

- A pain that doesn't go away
- New lumps, bumps, swellings, rashes, bruises, or bleeding
- Appetite changes, nausea, vomiting, diarrhea, or constipation
- Weight loss that you can't explain
- A fever, cough, or hoarseness that does not go away
- Any other symptoms that worry you

> **THE QUESTION DOCTOR SAYS:**
>
> When you are asking the Magic Question for chemotherapy, be sure to phrase your question, "How clear-cut is my case . . ." rather than "Is my case clear-cut?" You'll learn a lot more from the answer to the first version of this question, which is an open-ended question, than from the yes/no response you'll get from the second version.

When in doubt, err on the side of asking your doctor rather than hesitating to call.

10. What can I do to minimize the side effects and stay healthy during my chemotherapy?

You need to take a proactive role in your own health care for maximum recovery and well-being. Asking this question helps to signal your good intentions and asks your doctor for her partnership.

It will take your body a lot of energy to heal during chemotherapy. It's important that you eat enough calories and protein and keep your weight stable. Your appetite may be affected by the drugs. Ask your doctor or nurse about a special diet while you are getting chemotherapy.

You won't know your own reactions and side effects until after you start chemotherapy. The National Cancer Institute's online publication, *Chemotherapy and You,* has detailed information to help you. It's available free of charge at www.cancer.gov, or call 1-800-4-CANCER (1-800-422-6237).

❯ The Magic Question

How clear-cut is my case for recommending chemotherapy treatment?

If your doctor indicates any degree of fuzziness or doubt, ask this follow-up question: "Have you discussed the use of chemotherapy

somewhat."

Second, the answer may reveal your doctor's bias for one treatment option over another. For example, some doctors prefer to do mastectomies instead of breast-sparing procedures because that's what they learned in medical school. The same is true with other standard treatments. Your doctor might just be in the habit of prescribing chemotherapy for the majority of her patients, without giving it much reflection.

This question is not meant to devalue the benefits of chemotherapy or challenge your doctor's judgment, but rather as a final check that you are indeed a good candidate for this often difficult and joyless treatment. No one should agree to chemotherapy without first fully understanding her other options.

Preferably, your doctor does participate in regular tumor team meetings as described on page 25. This is a quality check to know that someone else is looking over your doctor's shoulder, each breast cancer patient is being treated individually, and your other treatment options have been fully reviewed. As Anna Nowak, M.D., a board-certified medical oncologist in Perth, Western Australia, observes, "To go to a cancer clinic or center where the doctors participate in a tumor board I think is very important from a patient's perspective."

CONCLUSION

Dr. Susan Love suggests this question to ask yourself as you weigh the pros and cons of having chemotherapy (or any other cancer treatment). She says, "Ask yourself, 'How would I feel if the cancer came back again in ten years and I had *not* had chemotherapy?' Then ask yourself, 'How would I feel if the cancer came back again in ten years and I had had chemo?' "

Oncologist Jennifer Armstrong, M.D., says, "Some of my patients didn't know what to do until they asked themselves what they would regret if they didn't do it [chemotherapy]."

You are not alone. No one deserves to get breast cancer. But everyone deserves the right to fight it.

THE 10 BEST RESOURCES

Adjuvant! Online. www.adjuvantonline.com/index.jsp.

American Cancer Society. "Understanding Chemotherapy: A Guide for Patients and Families." www.cancer.org/docroot/ETO/ETO_1_5x_ Guide_for_Patient_and_Families.asp.

Breastcancer.org. "Chemotherapy." www.breastcancer.org/treatment/che motherapy/index.jsp.

Cancer Treatment Centers of America. "Chemotherapy." www.cancercen ter.com/conventional-cancer-treatment/chemotherapy.cfm.

Lyss, Alan P., Humberto Fagundes, and Patricia Corrigan. *Chemotherapy and Radiation For Dummies.* Hoboken, NJ: Wiley, 2005.

Mayo Clinic. "Chemotherapy—Treatment Options at Mayo Clinic." www.mayoclinic.org/chemotherapy/.

McKay, Judith, and Nancee Hirano. *The Chemotherapy & Radiation Therapy Survival Guide*, 2nd ed. Oakland, CA: New Harbinger Publications, 1998.

Medicine.net. "Chemotherapy: Treatment and Side Effects

... radiotherapy) is the careful use of high-energy radiation to kill cancer cells and stop them from spreading. It destroys the cancer cells' ability to reproduce or grow. Radiation therapy doesn't kill cancer cells right away. This is why it often takes days or weeks of frequent treatments. It is a local therapy, meaning that it affects cancer cells only in the area where the radiation is directed.

If you have radiation therapy, you'll be under the care of a radiation oncologist, who is a specialist in using radiation therapy to treat cancer. He will meet with you in advance to explain the radiation therapy procedures, your dosage, treatment plan, ways to minimize side effects, and what to expect at follow-up visits. This doctor will work closely with your medical oncologist, surgeon, nurse, and the others on your medical team to plan your treatments, assess how well the radiation has worked, and check for side effects. Radiation therapy is often used after breast-conserving surgery. Other times, radiation therapy beforehand can minimize the need for radical surgery. The timing for radiation therapy is important if you are considering reconstructive breast surgery.

For women with breast cancer, radiation therapy is often only part of their treatment. Radiation therapy is often used with other cancer treatments, including breast surgery, chemotherapy, and hormone therapy. You doctor may decide to use radiation therapy either before or after your surgery or in conjunction with chemotherapy.

>>>THE 10 BEST QUESTIONS
About Radiation Therapy

1. What is the precise intent of this proposed radiation therapy and what kind will I be given?

As with chemotherapy, there are three basic reasons for radiation therapy. These are to:

1. Cure the cancer
2. Stop the cancer
3. Slow the growth of the cancer, relieve symptoms, or pain, or reduce pressure

The best of all, of course, is to be completely cured and cancer free. Your doctors may think that radiation therapy before or after surgery can shrink your tumor to the point that it's unlikely to recur. In the third scenario, radiation therapy can slow down metastatic disease for a tumor that has spread or grown. Radiation therapy is also used to relieve symptoms or pain or reduce pressure.

There are three types of radiation therapy that your doctor may recommend for treatment:

1. **External beam therapy** is a method for targeting and delivering a beam of high-energy X-rays to the location of the tumor. The radiation oncologist should use careful planning to protect the surrounding tissues.

2. **Intensity-modulated radiation therapy (IMRT)** is an advanced method that uses computers to deliver precisely controlled radiation doses to specific tumor areas. Treatment is carefully planned using three-dimensional (3D) computerized tomography (CT) images that help determine dosages based on the tumor's shape.

THE QUESTION DOCTOR

3. **Interstitial therapy** (or **brachytherapy**) is an internal radiation therapy that involves the temporary placement of radioactive materials within your breast. This type of radiation therapy gives you a boost of radiation in a higher dose and in a shorter time than external radiation.

If you have a choice, some radiation oncologists would recommend IMRT. Higher and more effective radiation doses can safely be delivered more precisely to your cancer cells with fewer side effects as compared with conventional radiation therapy techniques.

However, IMRT isn't a magic bullet. As Albert L. Blumberg, M.D., radiation oncologist and vice chair of the Department of Radiation Oncology at the Greater Baltimore Medical Center in Baltimore, Maryland, says, "If there was one obvious right answer, everyone would be doing it and everyone would be treated the same."

2. What percentage of improvement can I reasonably expect from this treatment?

The best answer to this question gives you both a percentage of improvement and an absolute number. Your medical oncologist or radiation oncologist should present you with this information.

If you want to know more, go to the Web site Adjuvant! Online (www.adjuvantonline.com). As mentioned earlier, this is a widely referenced source that helps health professionals and patients with early cancer understand the benefits, risks, and statistical data of different therapies.

3. What short-term side effects are possible? How will you help me to manage these side effects?

Radiation doesn't hurt while it's being given, but many people experience side effects or discomfort from its cumulative effects on their bodies over time. Side effects occur because the high doses of radiation used to kill your cancer cells can also kill your healthy cells.

Many women experience side effects such as skin problems, fluid buildup (called lymphedema), and fatigue. These side effects gradually disappear once your treatments are finished. The acute tiredness may continue for some months.

Your skin may look red, irritated, sunburned, or tanned in the treatment area. After a few weeks, your skin may be dry or reddened. The good news is that these skin changes most likely will go away in a month or two after you finish radiation therapy.

Let your doctors know about any side effects you experience. Ask for their help in resolving them; they may suggest mild soaps or provide guidelines for sun exposure.

With more serious side effects, ask what medications might help to relieve your discomfort.

4. What long-term side effects are possible? How will you help me to manage these side effects? Are there any side effects that may not go away?

A common long-term side effect is fatigue or feeling physically, mentally, and emotionally tired. You have less energy for your normal routines. Cancer fatigue is different from temporary daily tiredness and can last a long time.

Some women experience side effects, including breast soreness

buildup. Rarely, the radiation may leave small red marks on the skin due to tiny broken blood vessels. For many women, however, the overall appearance of the breast is unchanged.

Other side effects can include breathlessness (due to the effect of radiation on the lung), heart damage, bone damage, and a weakening of the ribs in the treatment area. When radiation treatments include the chest area, the lungs can be affected and cause fibrosis (lung stiffening or scarring). However, these side effects are very rare. Be sure to tell your doctor if you experience shortness of breath at any time during or after your radiation therapy.

Be sure to ask the last part of this Best Question. Don't assume that your side effects will finally go away forever. They may or may not. Insist that your doctor be fully candid with you about possible permanent changes from the radiation. Keep your doctor informed about your side effects at all times.

5. How will my skin, heart, and other internal organs and healthy tissue be protected from the radiation's effects?

Radiation not only kills or slows the growth of cancer cells, but it also affects nearby healthy cells. The healthy cells almost always recover after treatment is over. However, because of the close proximity of your breast to your heart, lungs, and other vital organs, special precautions need to be taken. This is especially true if your left breast (over your heart) is affected.

The best answer to this question will include telling you that this radiation center or doctor uses the newest radiation techniques, such as IMRT and 3D conformal radiation therapy to allow higher doses of radiation aimed at your cancer while reducing the radiation's impact on nearby healthy tissue.

To spare normal tissues such as the skin surrounding your breast and your heart, shaped radiation beams are aimed from several angles to intersect at the tumor, providing a much larger absorbed dose there than in the surrounding, healthy tissue.

Two other ways that doctors try to protect your healthy tissue are by spreading the treatments over time, such as giving radiation in daily doses once a day for several weeks, and by using the lowest dose possible that will still be effective.

6. What is my overall treatment plan? How long will each session of radiation therapy take? How long will I be under treatment (number of days or weeks)?

Because there are many variables that determine which treatments are prescribed (your tumor's stage, size, location, aggressiveness, etc.), each woman's treatment plan will have a different schedule. Some women have radiation therapy before surgery to shrink the tumor, some women have radiation therapy after surgery to kill off remaining cancer cells, and other women have only radiation therapy. Still others have radiation therapy along with surgery, chemotherapy, and/or hormone therapy.

Radiation therapy does not kill cancer cells right away. This is why it often takes days or weeks of treatment. Treatment is normally given in the hospital radiation department as a series of short daily outpatient sessions (about ten to fifteen minutes each) Monday through Friday, with a rest on the weekends. A course of radiation therapy for breast cancer typically lasts from three to six weeks.

Understanding your total time commitment and total treat-

this best Question now will give you some sense of control over your already busy schedule.

7. How will my daily life be affected during and after treatments? Will I need someone to take care of me?

Most likely, your doctor can't answer this question directly because he doesn't really know what your daily life is like. But you do. Think for yourself, "How tired do I normally feel at the end of the day?" "Am I a sound sleeper or already stressed out or impossibly overextended?" These factors and others in your life will impact your personal reactions to radiation therapy.

You'll probably want to know now if you'll be too tired to work full time, care for your children, or keep up with your other normal responsibilities. Some women are able to work full time during radiation therapy. Others can only work part time or not at all. How much you are able to work depends on how you feel, your health-insurance coverage, and your employer's flexibility.

You are likely to feel well enough to work when you start radiation therapy. As time goes on, don't be surprised if you are more tired, have less energy, or feel weak. Once you have finished your treatment, it may take a few weeks or many months for you to feel better.

You may get to a point during your radiation therapy when you feel too weak to work. Talk with your employer about medical leave. Check with your health insurance provider on paying for

> I was surprised how tired I was after my radiation therapy. Some days I could barely get out of bed. My mom helped me with the kids and I felt a tremendous relief. My neighbor insisted on driving me to my appointments. At first I resisted, but then I was so glad to have her company.
>
> — MARIA, FORTY-THREE, MIAMI BEACH

treatments while you are on medical leave.

As with chemotherapy, you may need a part-time caregiver to help you while you are undergoing radiation therapy. This treatment is no joy ride (especially its cumulative effects near the end of the scheduled treatments), so build a good support system now to help you later.

8. What, if any, restrictions will there be on my normal activities while I'm undergoing treatment?

The American Cancer Society suggests you avoid putting anything hot or cold, such as heating pads or ice packs, on your treated skin, unless advised to by your doctor. Ditto for powders, creams, perfumes, deodorants, body oils, ointments, lotions, or home remedies. Many skin products can leave a coating on the skin that may cause irritation and could change how the radiation enters your body. Ask your doctor or nurse about using sunscreen lotions.

Also discuss with your doctor your lifestyle concerns (diet, exercise, work, etc.) as well as any complementary treatments. See chapter 12 on complementary medicine.

9. What symptoms or changes in my body are serious enough to warrant my calling you?

If you know in advance which symptoms after radiation therapy are considered normal and which ones aren't, you'll be more likely to pick up the phone with confidence when calling your doctor. Possible warning signs are aches or chest pains, rashes or skin burns, lymphedema (swelling in your arm), pain that doesn't go away, loss of strength, numbness ...

... can I do to minimize the side effects and stay healthy during radiation therapy?

Think proactively and let your doctor know you want to stay as physically fit as possible during your treatments. Get his best advice for coping with possible side effects, such as keeping your appetite and weight stable, and dealing with loss of appetite or fatigue.

Your doctor may suggest a special diet to help you with eating problems. He might also suggest you eliminate or minimize alcohol or certain foods during your radiation therapy. The American Cancer Society offers common-sense suggestions for eating problems on its Web site at www.cancer.org/docroot/MBC/MBC_6_1_when_treatment_causes_eating_problems.asp.

❯ The Magic Question

Do I have any special health or personal considerations that might be affected by radiation therapy?

This is a personal question targeted to your own medical history and personal needs. For example, if you have a history of heart disease, ask what special precautions the radiation oncologist will take in planning and administering your treatments.

Perhaps you enjoy playing the piano. If so, ask about how radiation therapy affects the nerves in the fingertips. This is a rare side effect in the general population, but if it happened to you, it might be extra difficult to cope with. Maybe you enjoy swimming and are concerned about how chlorinated water might affect the irradiated skin.

The point is to make sure your doctor assesses radiation treatment for you as a unique individual, including your prior medical issues and lifestyle. Your doctor should discuss the treatment pros and cons about you personally, not the statistically average breast cancer patient.

CONCLUSION

As with other breast cancer treatments, radiation therapy presents a mixed bag of benefits and risks for most patients. If your doctor suggests radiation therapy and recommends a radiation oncologist (radiation specialist) to you, use the 10 Best Questions in chapter 2 to ensure you've got a top doctor.

Then ask your new radiation oncologist the Best Questions in this chapter so you'll fully understand his rationale and your options for radiation therapy. Radiation oncologist Dr. Albert Blumberg says of his fellow doctors, "We need to give women the knowledge to make their decisions because at the end of the day there are no guarantees for a 100 percent cancer cure."

THE 10 BEST RESOURCES

Adjuvant! Online. "Adjuvant! FAQs." www.adjuvantonline.com/faq.jsp.

American Cancer Society. "Understanding Radiation Therapy: A Guide for Patients and Families." www.cancer.org/docroot/ETO/ETO_1_5x_radiation_therapy_guide_for_patients_and_families.asp.

American Society for Therapeutic Radiology and Oncology. "Welcome to RT [radiation therapy] Answers." www.rtanswers.org/.

Breastcancer.org. "Radiation Therapy." www.breastcancer.org/treatment/radiation/index.jsp.

Cukier, Daniel. *Coping with Ch...*

National Cancer Institute. "A Collection of Radiation Therapy Fact Sheets." www.cancer.gov/cancertopics/wtk/index.

National Cancer Institute. "Radiation Therapy and You: Support for People with Cancer." www.cancer.gov/cancertopics/radiation-therapy-and-you.

RadiologyInfo. "Breast Cancer." www.radiologyinfo.org/en/info.cfm?pg= breastcancer.

The female hormone estrogen blesses you with youthfulness, but it can also curse you with breast cancer. Hormones are substances that occur naturally in the body where they control the growth and activity of normal cells. Although they do not usually affect most cancer cells, in breast cancer the situation is different for some tumors.

Your ovaries are your body's main source of estrogen until menopause. After menopause, smaller amounts are still made in the body's fat tissue, where a hormone made by the adrenal glands is converted into estrogen. Estrogen promotes the growth of about two-thirds of breast cancers containing estrogen receptors (ER-positive cancers) and/or progesterone receptors (PR-positive cancers). This explains the need for hormone therapy, which blocks the effects of estrogen or lowers estrogen levels to treat ER-positive and PR-positive breast cancers.

Hormone therapy involves either drugs or surgery. The most common hormone therapy for early stage breast cancer is the drug tamoxifen. A newer class of drugs called aromatase inhibitors is also available exclusively for postmenopausal women. Surgical therapy involves the suppression or surgical removal of the ovaries, and even radiation therapy has been used in the past to suppress the ovaries.

Don't confuse the term "hormone therapy" for treating breast cancer and "hormone replacement therapy" or "HRT," which is typically used by postmenopausal women to treat symptoms like hot flashes. Hormone therapy for cancer treatment stops hormones from getting to cancer cells and thus prevents the cancer from growing. Hormone replacement therapy for postmenopausal women without cancer adds more hormones to a woman's body to counter the effects of menopause.

>>>THE 10 BEST QUESTIONS
About Hormone Therapy

1. What is hormone therapy and why do you think I'm a good candidate for it?

Ask your doctor to explain hormone therapy to you in terms that make it personal to your case of breast cancer.

Briefly, there are two kinds of hormone therapy:

1. Drugs that inhibit estrogen and progesterone from promoting breast cancer cell growth
2. Drugs or surgery to turn off the production of hormones from the ovaries

Hormone-therapy drugs prevent estrogen from binding to cells and act like an anti-estrogen. They help to reduce the risk of cancer recurrence after surgery and are frequently used for advanced or metastatic breast cancers. For women who are high-risk candidates for developing breast cancer, hormone therapy may be prescribed as a preventive measure.

Hormone therapy via drugs is a systemic therapy (affects your whole body). It is usually used as an adjuvant, or additional, therapy following the primary treatments of breast surgery, chemotherapy, and/or radiation therapy.

Most women with metastatic disease *and* positive hormone receptors are good candidates for hormone therapy. Sometimes pa-

tumor? What was the HER2/neu status?

During the diagnostic process, tests were done to determine if your cancer cells have estrogen or progesterone receptors. You should have received this information from your pathology report. See chapter 3 for a more complete explanation.

The clearest indication of your candidacy for hormone therapy is your hormone receptor status. If your tumor is not hormone sensitive, a hormone therapy is generally useless and potentially harmful. Hormonal therapies are only effective in women whose cancer cells have receptors (are sensitive) for estrogen and/or progesterone on their surface. This is known as being estrogen-receptor positive (ER+) or progesterone-receptor positive (PR+). Reviewing your hormone receptor status with your doctor is a key element in your discussion about hormone therapy.

According to Clifford Hudis, M.D., chief of the Breast Cancer Medicine Service at Memorial Sloan-Kettering Cancer Center in New York City, "Starting hormone therapy in the first year after breast cancer diagnosis and initial treatment is important."

3. What is the precise intent of the proposed hormone therapy?

The general objective of all hormone therapy is to block or remove the effects that your body's production of estrogen and progesterone is having on your cancer cells.

There are different types of hormone therapy, and each works slightly differently. The main treatment options are:

- Tamoxifen (see Best Question 4)
- Aromatase inhibitors (see Best Question 4)
- Zoladex and Lupron (see Best Question 4)
- Ovarian ablation (stopping the ovaries by surgical removal or radiation)

Here are some examples of how hormone therapies are used and why:

- Treatment of ductal carcinoma in situ (DCIS) along with breast-sparing surgery or mastectomy
- Adjuvant treatment of lobular carcinoma in situ (LCIS) to reduce the risk of developing more advanced breast cancer
- Adjuvant treatment of early stage invasive breast cancer in men and women whose cancers are estrogen-receptor positive
- Treatment of recurrent or metastatic breast cancer
- To prevent breast cancer in women at high risk for developing breast cancer

Each hormone therapy treatment plan and its objectives are as unique as each case of breast cancer. What you want to understand is your doctor's rationale in prescribing it for *you*.

4. What drugs will I be given? Is there a generic form? Is the generic form as effective as the name brand?

There are three categories of hormone therapy drugs and the most common types for each are:

- **Tamoxifen (also called Nolvadex).** Tamoxifen has been the most widely prescribed and successful anti-estrogen therapy for breast cancer for more than twenty-five years. This anti-estrogen drug works by preventing

- **Aromatase inhibitors, also called anastrozole (Arimidex), letrozole (Femara), and exemestane (Aromasin).** Recently a new group of hormone therapy drugs, the aromatase inhibitors, has been developed that block estrogen from being made in the tissues of postmenopausal women. Aromatase inhibitors are used only in postmenopausal women. Research has shown that for some women, taking aromatase inhibitors instead of tamoxifen, or after a period of tamoxifen treatment, can further reduce the chance of their cancer coming back. An important consideration when choosing among different drugs is your pre- or postmenopausal status. The clearest indication of whether a woman should take tamoxifen or an aromatase inhibitor is her menstrual status. Prior to menopause, with most estrogen coming directly from the ovaries, aromatase inhibitors are insufficient to suppress natural estrogen, and tamoxifen will work best.

- **Pituitary down-regulators, also called Zoladex, or goserelin, and Lupron (leuprolide).** Pituitary down-regulators reduce the production of estrogen-stimulating hormones by the brain. The result for premenopausal women is a lower level of estrogen along with temporary infertility. This type of therapy is given as a monthly injection.

See more discussion on these drugs in the following Best Questions.

5. What benefits can I reasonably expect from this treatment?

According to both the American Cancer Society and the National Cancer Institute, the benefits of tamoxifen as a treatment for breast cancer are firmly established and far outweigh the potential risks. Tamoxifen helps prevent the original breast cancer from returning as well as preventing the development of new cancers in your other breast.

The National Cancer Institute funded a large study in 1998 to determine whether tamoxifen would reduce the occurrence of breast cancer in healthy women known to be at high risk. The results of the trial showed a 50-percent reduction in both invasive and noninvasive breast cancer in the treated women. A 2004 review by the Cochrane Collaboration concluded that taking tamoxifen can greatly improve survival rates of women with ER-positive breast cancer.

While tamoxifen blocks estrogen in breast tissue, it acts like estrogen in other tissue. This means that women who take tamoxifen may derive many of the beneficial effects of postmenopausal estrogen replacement therapy (HRT), such as lower blood cholesterol and slower bone loss which helps prevent osteoporosis.

For many postmenopausal women it is helpful to have an aromatase inhibitor as part of hormonal therapy treatment for early breast cancer. Hormone therapy in general is safe and has relatively few serious side effects. Discuss the benefits of hormone therapy in your specific case with your doctor.

6. What short-term side effects and risks are possible? What can you do to help me manage them?

All types of hormone therapies have potential short-term mild to moderate side effects. Any of these treatments can mimic the troublesome side effects of menopause, including fatigue, hot flashes, vaginal discomfort, fluid retention, weight gain, irregular periods, reduced sexual drive, nausea, ...

... symptoms described above.

Zoladex actually brings on a temporary menopause. So again, you may be stuck with hot flashes as your ovaries temporarily shut down until you are off the Zoladex.

Discuss your specific concerns about short-term side effects with your doctor. Ask for his assistance to alleviate bothersome side effects, as well as for advice on what you might be able to do pro-actively (diet, exercise, and lifestyle changes). Memorial Sloan-Kettering's Dr. Clifford Hudis summarizes, "The side effects of hormone therapy can be annoying, but they aren't usually danger-ous or life-threatening."

7. What long-term side effects and risks are possible? What can you do to help me manage these side effects and risks? Are there any side effects that may not go away?

Rare but serious side effects are possible. The key to this question is to make sure you don't skip the last part of it: "Are there any side effects that may not go away?" Long-term side effects that are re-versible are not as serious as ones that will never go away.

Tamoxifen may slightly increase your risk for blood clots in your legs or lungs, strokes, uterine cancer, endometrial cancer, and cataracts. A forty-year clinical trial run by the National Surgical Adjuvant Breast and Bowel Project (NSABP) and the National Cancer Institute found endometrial cancer occurred 2.5 times more frequently in women taking tamoxifen.

Fertility is affected by tamoxifen (you become more fertile). If you are premenopausal, discuss birth control and pregnancy issues with your doctor. Women are advised not to become pregnant while taking hormone therapy.

Unlike tamoxifen, aromatase inhibitors don't increase the risk of blood clots and strokes. However, because they have only been used for a few years, the long-term side effects of aromatase inhibitors aren't fully known yet. Taking aromatase inhibitors over the long term may make your bones more fragile. Ask about regular bone density tests and preventive measures you can take, such as getting prescriptions for calcium and vitamin D supplements.

If you have your ovaries removed, you will no longer be able to have children. If you take Zoladex, your infertility is potentially reversible, unless you were borderline menopausal anyway. If so, your body may begin its natural cycle of shifting into menopause earlier than it would have without the hormone therapy.

An example of additional medical care you might need while taking hormone therapy is to have extra gynecologic surveillance, such as screening for uterine cancer or ovarian cysts or having bone density tests.

Discuss your specific concerns with your doctor and have her review your personal medical history. If you are planning a future pregnancy, make sure you understand how hormone therapy might affect you. Ask for advice and assistance.

8. How does hormone therapy fit into my overall treatment plan? Will I be given the hormone therapy along with other forms of treatment?

This is the "big picture" question to help you understand your doctor's master treatment plan for you. Understanding the answer to this question will help you plot out the logistics of your cancer recovery and how hormone therapy may affect your everyday life.

breast before surgery. This means you will need a less invasive operation.

The most common treatment plan starts with an initial surgery (a lumpectomy or mastectomy and possible breast reconstruction), chemotherapy, and radiation therapy. Hormone therapy is usually started after chemotherapy.

9. How soon before or after surgery should I start hormone therapy? How long will I be on the therapy?

In general, starting hormone therapy in the first year after a breast cancer diagnosis is important. But this is not a cut-and-dried decision, and there's currently debate in the medical community about the timing of these drugs. Drug manufacturers put marketing pressure on oncologists and may give them conflicting or profit-driven information in an attempt to sell more of their drugs faster. Ask your doctor for the rationale behind his recommendation for your individualized care.

Many women take tamoxifen for five years after they are first diagnosed with early stage breast cancer and have surgery. The optimal length of treatment with aromatase inhibitors has not yet been determined. Patients with advanced breast cancer may take tamoxifen for varying lengths of time, depending on their response to this treatment and other factors.

PREMENOPAUSAL WOMEN AND HORMONE THERAPY

According to Dr. Clifford Hudis, if you are premenopausal, ask for your doctor's views and advice on these two additional Best Questions:

> "Is there a role for ovarian suppression in my case?" This is potentially controversial because breast cancer specialists still aren't sure of the value of this treatment plan.

> If you want to get pregnant later (or at least not lose your options), ask, "What's the likely impact of hormone therapy on my ability to have children later?" If you take tamoxifen for five years (the standard treatment) you may be beyond normal childbearing age by the time it would be safe for you to get pregnant.

10. How will hormone therapy affect my risk for a local recurrence, distant metastasis, or a new breast cancer?

A local recurrence means the cancer comes back to the same breast. Distant metastasis is a cancer that shows up in a part of your body other than your breast, like your liver. An example of a new breast cancer is the presence of cancer cells in the other breast.

Research studies have concluded that when tamoxifen is taken for five years for early stage breast cancer it reduces the risk of recurrence of the original cancer by about 50 percent. Tamoxifen also reduces the risk of developing new cancers in the other breast.

Recent clinical trials compared how well tamoxifen and aromatase inhibitors prevented recurrence or metastatic cancer. Early results indicate some advantages of aromatase inhibitors with certain types of breast cancer, but it's best to check with your doctor to understand the details of your case and her treatment preferences for you.

...menopausal status. If you are postmenopausal you may be a candidate for aromatase inhibitors following tamoxifen treatment or as an alternative to tamoxifen.

Sometimes your menopausal status is clear, but sometimes it's not. The definition of menopause is typically one year with no period and no reason (pregnancy) for no period. But if you are premenopausal or going through chemotherapy, deciding your status can become surprisingly difficult.

As Dr. Clifford Hudis explains: "For example, you are forty-nine years old and you are currently undergoing chemotherapy. You had your last period in the second week of the chemotherapy program and have had hot flashes and other menopausal symptoms. Now it's four months later and you are finishing chemotherapy. Your doctor is getting ready to discuss hormone therapy with you. You are not by definition postmenopausal. But you may appear to be postmenopausal in a superficial way."

Your doctor may be willing to gamble that you are postmenopausal. If so, ask him to look up which of the aromatase inhibitors clinical trials you would actually have been eligible for. You don't want your doctor to guess whether your ovaries are still working. You risk reduced drug effectiveness and even possibly taking the drug during a pregnancy.

Or your doctor, especially if he is not a breast cancer specialist, may not know enough about hormone therapy even to question this distinction. It may be up to you to open this discussion. Let your doctor reassure you that this is a factor that he has already taken into consideration when planning your treatment.

CONCLUSION

The benefits of hormone therapy in reducing the chance of the breast cancer coming back far outweigh the risks of side effects for most women. However, there are no absolute guidelines and no guarantees. The newest research keeps changing our standards for the best practices to follow.

At many levels, researchers are just now starting to understand how hormone therapies really work. Some older drugs or treatments can turn out to be just as good, cheaper, or even better than the new treatments being tested in current studies.

THE 10 BEST RESOURCES

Adjuvant! Online. "Hormone Therapy." www.adjuvantonline.com/index.jsp.

Allen, Jane E. "Everything You Need to Know About Aromatase Inhibitors." *MAMM Magazine*, July–August 2005. www.mamm.com.

American Cancer Society. "Detailed Guide: Breast Cancer: Hormone Therapy." www.cancer.org/docroot/CRI/content/CRI_2_4_4X_Hormone_Therapy_5.asp?sitearea=.

The Cochrane Collaboration. "Long Term Hormone Therapy for Perimenopausal and Postmenopausal Women." www.cochrane.org/reviews/en/ab004143.html.

Love, Susan, Karen Lindsey, and Marcia Williams. "Treatment Options: Hormone Therapy," in *Dr. Susan Love's Breast Book,* 4th ed. Cambridge: Da Capo Press, 2005.

Memorial Sloan-Kettering Cancer Center. "Systemic Therapy." www.mskcc.org/mskcc/html/2380.cfm.

National Cancer Institute. "A

National Cancer Institute. "Fact Sheet: Tamoxifen: Questions and Answers." www.cancer.gov/cancertopics/factsheet/Therapy/tamoxifen.

standpoint of receiving a high level of care and in helping develop the latest products to treat debilitating or life-threatening diseases.

—Dr. C. Everett Koop,
former U.S. Surgeon General

A **clinical trial** is a research program conducted with patients to evaluate a new medical treatment, drug, or device. The purpose of a breast cancer clinical trial is to find new and improved methods of treating the disease.

Clinical trials make it possible to apply the latest scientific and technological advances to patient care. During a breast cancer clinical trial, researchers, usually doctors, use the best available treatment as a standard to evaluate a new treatment. The new treatment may be a new drug, surgical technique, radiation dosage, or a complementary medicine.

From a patient's perspective, the benefits of participating in a clinical trial include:

- Increased patient monitoring and surveillance by the health-care team that may not be normally given with standard care

- Health-care benefits, such as free examinations to assess the risks of breast cancer among the participant's female family members or a free gym membership

- Long-term information and better care for a family member, such as a sister, daughter, or niece who may potentially be at risk for breast cancer, too

In 2004, more than 17 million people inquired about participating in clinical trials in the United States, and more than 2 million people volunteered for industry- and government-sponsored studies. The growing number of participants in clinical trials indicates a trend toward patients being more receptive to participating in clinical trials (also called "investigational treatments") as one of their medical options.

More than eighty thousand clinical trials (covering all diseases) are conducted in the United States annually. A clinical trial can be an excellent opportunity for patients to find promising new treatments. However, even though the majority of clinical trials are safe and effective, there are risks for volunteers. A 2002 CenterWatch analysis of Food and Drug Administration (FDA) data found that one in thirty volunteers typically experiences a serious side effect, and one in ten thousand dies as the result of the effects of the study drug.

The number of women with breast cancer who participate in clinical trials is small; Dr. Susan Love, breast surgeon and specialist, estimates the total at only about 5 percent. Dr. Love says, "I don't think it comes up as much as it should. Most physicians don't offer clinical trials to their patients. I would say 90 percent don't."

According to a 2002 study by CenterWatch, a Boston-based publisher of clinical trial information, the majority of people (70 percent) who enter clinical trials do so without knowing what questions to ask. Many people reported that they didn't understand the risks of study participation, and 10 percent of volunteers admitted they didn't even look at the informed consent form before signing it.

... chapter, along with your own questions, so you can fully understand what you're getting into.

This chapter also includes a brief description of **genetic therapy**, a therapy that is currently only being studied in clinical trials with nonhuman subjects. There are no Best Questions for genetic therapy because it's only in the experimental stage. It's included here because of all the press about genetic therapies that might lead you to wonder about its availability and use in your case.

〉〉〉THE 10 BEST QUESTIONS
Before Participating in a Clinical Trial

1. How will this trial help me personally?

Keep this conversation at the personal level—benefits for you personally—rather than generic or statistical facts. Your essential question is, "What's in it for me?" Be sure you understand your doctor's comparison of your treatment plan versus the treatments you'd receive as a participant in a clinical trial.

The possible benefits of clinical trials are:

- High-quality cancer care.
- Access to new treatments, drugs, or devices.
- You take an active role in your health care.
- Most participants receive careful monitoring during the trial.

- You have the chance to help other women and improve cancer treatment.

The possible drawbacks are:

- New treatments under study are not always better or even as good as standard treatments.
- It may not work for you.
- You may be randomly assigned to the standard treatment instead of the new treatment, thus missing out on the new treatment while going to the extra trouble of being in the trial.
- Your health insurance carrier may not cover all your costs in the study.
- Some trials are time-consuming or disruptive to daily routines.

Dr. Bruce J. Hillman, a professor of radiology at the University of Virginia and a ten-year veteran of leading National Cancer Institute clinical trials, comments, "The bias for patients is that the newest treatment is the better treatment, but that's not always true."

2. What are the researchers hoping to learn from this study? What phase is this trial?

Clinical trials are developed for different reasons. Some study the effectiveness of certain drugs, while others study which doses are safe. Know the purpose of the study prior to signing on.

A key follow-up question is to ask, "What phase is this trial?" Clinical trials are usually conducted in a series of steps, called Phase I, Phase II, Phase III, and Phase IV trials. Treatment clinical trials listed in PDQ, the National Cancer Institute's comprehensive cancer information database, are always assigned a phase.

Phase I trials usually enroll

... . study the effectiveness of a drug or treatment. They usually focus on a particular type of cancer with a small number of participants. There are strict eligibility requirements. The goal of Phase II trials is to establish that a new treatment substantially benefits at least 20 percent of patients who receive the drug. The trial also confirms that the dose chosen in Phase I trials is indeed safe.

Phase III trials provide hard, statistical evidence about whether a drug prolongs survival or improves quality of life, and these trials involve large groups of patients. The new drug or combination is compared to the best current treatment for a particular kind of cancer. Testing may involve hundreds or thousands of people over as many as five years. These studies use a "randomized control group," which means some volunteers get the standard treatment (the control group) and others get the drug being tested. This removes bias in reporting results because patients don't know in advance which group they are in. Many randomized studies consist of the standard treatment plus an additional treatment or drug. Sometimes this combination (standard treatment plus experimental treatment) is better for patients and other times it is not. This comparison is the whole point of doing a clinical trial.

Phase IV trials further evaluate the long-term safety and effectiveness of a treatment, usually take place after a treatment has been approved for standard use, and involve hundreds or thousands of people.

It's important to note that due to the serious nature of cancer, there are no placebos (fake drugs) used in cancer clinical trials. This means that you can rest assured that you will be getting at minimum the current standard treatment.

3. Who is sponsoring this trial? Describe this trial's prior history and measurable outcomes.

This is an important question because it will help you understand more about the researchers' motives. The gold standard in clinical trials is sponsorship by a highly respected group such as the National Cancer Institute (NCI) or one of the NCI designated Cancer Centers. Drug companies can also offer solid and ethical trials. By understanding the trial's sponsors, you'll start to have clues into their possible biases. See the Magic Question™ below, which expands on this issue.

Learn everything you can about the study's previous history. Some of what you can learn will be determined by what phase this particular clinical trial is in. If there is a history, ask about the previous results, success rates, and the number of people involved. Get the details on how the study is being conducted, what specifically is asked of participants (such as being hospitalized or taking new drugs), and any additional tests or biopsies that will be asked of you. Ask the "who, what, when, where, and why" questions to prompt a full explanation from your doctor. Find out if you'll be required to switch doctors or cancer care centers. Another important consideration is stability. You don't necessarily want to be seen by a series of rotating doctors, each one representing another "get acquainted" chore for you.

AM I RIGHT FOR A CLINICAL TRIAL?

... for taking

... have the time needed to participate in a clinical trial? Some clinical trials are time-consuming and may take years, while others are much shorter.

4. **How important is it to me that I work with my current oncologist?** If your current oncologist is not part of the clinical trial, you may need to find a new doctor who is.

5. **Am I confident and comfortable with the goals of this study and with the staff at the research center?** Ideally, the trial's goals match your personal values and the staff will treat you well.

6. **How important is it to me to help other women with breast cancer?** Participating in a clinical trial is a way of helping future generations of breast cancer patients, if this is your thing.

7. **How will this trial affect my daily life?** Logistical concerns include travel time and expenses, child care needs, and time off from work.

8. **Will my family and loved ones support my decision to participate in this clinical trial?** Talk over your interests and the clinical trial's requirements with the other people in your life who might be affected.

9. **Have I read the informed consent document and taken enough time to truly understand it? Has everything been adequately explained to me?** Doctors and nurses will definitely answer your questions about the informed consent documents, so be sure to ask about anything that's unclear to you.

10. **How realistic am I about what I have to gain personally from participating?** Don't answer this question in a vacuum of knowledge about the trial that you are considering.

4. What are the possible risks and complications, both short term and long term, in my case?

Make the focus of this answer about you and your own type of breast cancer, rather than general statistics that mean less to you personally. Be sure your doctor tells you as much as is known about possible long-term residual effects from taking an experimental drug or treatment.

A really smart follow-up question in this discussion is, "What *don't* we know yet about this new drug or treatment?" This question will encourage your doctor to reveal candidly any design flaws and possible side effects. It's quite possible that there are many unknowns because of the experimental nature of clinical trials, or perhaps your doctor may not be fully informed about this particular trial.

5. What safety measures are built into this study?

You want to understand how this study maximizes your potential benefits while minimizing potential harm. Your doctor's answer to this question should include detailed information about how patient safety will be monitored and a description of patient safeguards. Ask, "Has this study been approved by an institutional review board (ethical panels comprised of doctors and other medical experts who work with the Food and Drug Administration)?" and "Did the review board that approved this trial have any ethical concerns with the trial?"

6. How long does this trial last? Where is it being conducted?

The length of clinical trials varies greatly, as does the amount of time required of you on a daily, weekly, or monthly basis. Sometimes trials involve one day or one blood draw. Often, especially in drug trials, the trial will last for several months or even years. Know the expected duration of your trial before signing on. Be sure to

find out the total time the trial will last (in m...
ask. "How ...

...kind of support will I receive during the trial?

Find out in advance what your insurance carrier will cover if you participate in this clinical trial, including costs out of your own pocket. Don't forget incidental costs, like additional child care or transportation costs, which can add up over time. You want to be compensated for your time and inconvenience by either your insurance carrier or the study's sponsors. Trials often pay for the doctors' visits, medications, blood work, or diagnostic tests that are part of the study. Know exactly who pays what and if you are getting paid before you sign anything.

You also want to know the details of how your health and well-being will be monitored during the trial. Find out if there's a system of checks and balances in place for any problems that occur during the trial. Ask if you'll be allowed to move from the standard treatment group to the experimental one if the new drug is clearly superior.

Ask the following questions:

- Who will be my medical team?
- Who can I call if I have questions?
- Who will be in charge of my care during the trial, especially if I experience side effects?
- Can I join support groups or talk about this trial if I want to?

- Will there be support for my family during the trial?
- How will my medical records and confidentiality be protected?

8. What will happen when the trial ends?

A key issue for you personally is to understand what kind (if any) of follow-up medical support will be there after the trial ends. Can you expect to receive medical care or some other kind of support follow-up care? Ask, "Will I have any posttrial responsibilities?" and "Who will be responsible for the posttrial segment of this study?" Sometimes the new drug or treatment is so useful that participants want to continue with it even after the trial ends. Find out if this will be an option for you. Ask, "Can I opt to remain on this treatment even after termination of the trial?" Last, you probably will want to know about how the study turned out. Find out how you will get the results at the trial's conclusion.

9. What happens if I'm harmed by the trial? Am I free to withdraw at any time without penalty?

Don't neglect to examine the worst-case scenario about patient safety. Ask the following questions:

- What will happen if I have complications as the result of this study?
- Who will be responsible?
- How will the trial sponsors be held accountable?
- Who will pay for my medical expenses if I'm injured?

You also want to know the details about leaving the study early, either by your choice or if you are asked to leave. If you leave early, find out if you'll have to seek treatment elsewhere and if there will be any restrictions on your future treatments.

Researchers do everything in their power to make certain you

THE QUESTION DOCTOR SAYS

...example, there may be a change in your health status that makes it dangerous for you to participate, or you may be unable to follow the prescribed protocol. Ask about the conditions and provisions for withdrawal. Your informed consent form should spell out an escape clause.

10. Am I a good candidate? Why or why not? What is your recommendation?

Ask your doctor to summarize your discussion with her about clinical trials by finding out if you are a good candidate, both from a medical perspective and in terms of eligibility. Stay alert to any possible bias on your doctor's part due to her own participation in a certain trial. You can phrase the question something like, "If you weren't doing this research, what would you say is best for me?" If you feel pressured to participate, go get an objective second opinion from a doctor not connected to this doctor or to the trial. See chapter 5 on second opinions.

❯ The Magic Question

Are there any other things I need to know about why the researchers are recruiting volunteers for this clinical trial? If you don't know, how can I find out more?

Doctors and research centers recommend specific clinical trials for a variety of reasons. While the vast majority of reasons involve purely

THE STORY ON GENE THERAPY AND CLINICAL TRIALS

Gene therapy is an experimental technique that uses genes to treat or prevent disease. In the future, this technique may allow doctors to treat a disorder by inserting a healthy gene into a patient's cells instead of using drugs or surgery.

Current research is examining several approaches to gene therapy, including:

> Replacing a mutated, diseased gene with a healthy copy of the gene

> Turning off a dysfunctional mutated gene

> Introducing a new gene into the body to help fight a disease like breast cancer

Although gene therapy is a promising treatment, this technique is still experimental, risky, and *not* yet available, only through a clinical trial basis. Edith Perez, M.D., a professor of medicine at the Mayo Clinic in Jacksonville, Florida, is researching the future promise of gene therapy for breast cancer. Dr. Perez says, "Gene therapy is far from being a reality for patients. The gene therapy approach, although theoretically very appealing, doesn't translate yet into therapy for patients. It's just pie in the sky right now."

For more information on gene therapy, see the National Cancer Institute's fact sheet, "Gene Therapy for Cancer: Questions and Answers" (www.cancer.gov/cancertopics/factsheet/therapy/gene).

humanitarian and scientific interests, there are a few rare exceptions. Some trials have trouble attracting enough participants and have to advertise to recruit volunteers. Find out specifically why there haven't been enough volunteers before you commit to a trial. It could be that the trial simply requires more participants than an individual researcher or cancer center can provide, or there could be other factors like a long-time commitment required from volunteers. This is your "better safe than sorry" question before participating in a clinical trial.

cruitment, Retention, and Outreach Core facility at the Abramson Cancer Center. She summarizes clinical trials with these comments: "Today's evidence-based treatments were yesterday's clinical trials. If you feel comfortable that your doctor is giving you the best evidence-based treatment, it's because someone did a clinical trial to be sure the treatment they are getting is actually effective."

THE 10 BEST RESOURCES

American Cancer Society. "Clinical Trials: What You Need to Know." www.cancer.org/docroot/ETO/content/ETO_6_3_Clinical_Trials_-_Patient_Participation.asp.

Centerwatch. Clinical trials listing service. www.centerwatch.com.

ClinicalTrials.gov. Registry of federally and privately supported clinical trials.

ClinicalTrials.gov. "Understanding Clinical Trials." www.clinicaltrials.gov/ct2/info/understand.

Coalition of Cancer Cooperative Groups. "TrialCheck." www.trialcheck.org/services/.

ECRI Institute. "Should I Enter a Clinical Trial? A Patient Reference Guide for Adults with a Serious or Life-Threatening Illness." www.ecri.org/Documents/Clinical_Trials_Patient_Reference_Guide.pdf.

Getz, Ken, and Deborah Borfitz. *Informed Consent: The Consumer's Guide to the Risks and Benefits of Volunteering for Clinical Trials*. Boston: Center-Watch, 2002.

National Cancer Institute. "Clinical Trials for Breast Cancer." www.cancer.gov/search/ResultsClinicalTrials.aspx?protocolsearchid=4284215.

National Cancer Institute. "Search for Clinical Trials." www.cancer.gov/clinicaltrials/search.

National Cancer Institute. "Taking Part in Cancer Treatment Research Studies." www.cancer.gov/clinicaltrials/Taking-Part-in-Cancer-Treatment-Research-Studies.

what comes up, when you sit in that silence. "Mama keeps whites bright like the sunlight; Mama's got the magic of Clorox 2."

—Ellen DeGeneres,
comedian

Complementary and alternative medicine (often called "CAM") is a group of diverse medical practices outside the boundaries of conventional medicine. With conventional medicine, the doctors have medical degrees (M.D.s), and others they work with belong to other fully accredited medical specializations, such as registered nurses or psychologists, and have attended advanced training at accredited institutions.

It's important to know that the terms "complementary" and "alternative" are often confused and used interchangeably. In fact, they have very different meanings and implications for your health care. **Alternative medicine** is treatment used *instead of* conventional medicine. **Complementary medicine** is used *together with* conventional medicine.

As Barrie Cassileth, Ph.D., the head of the Integrative Medicine Service at the Memorial Sloan-Kettering Cancer Center in New York, explains, "Alternative therapies represent a tremendous economic boom for people who are selling total nonsense. These are usually bogus therapies that have been studied and found not to work or have not been studied at all because they're nonsensical and unworthy of the time and cost that research requires. But the market is enormous and some people make a very good living in selling quackery."

Stephen Barrett, M.D., founder of the medical consumer watchdog Web site Quackwatch, agrees: "If you are trying to find an alternative method that influences the course of your cancer, there aren't any and it's an absolute waste of time."

In other words, forget alternative medicine for your cancer care! There are *no* viable alternatives to mainstream, conventional medicine for fighting cancer. Please don't abandon your regular cancer treatments in favor of an alternative or complementary treatment only.

In contrast, complementary therapies are often used along with mainstream cancer care. Complementary medicine can be very useful, but it doesn't kill cancer; it only controls the symptoms. It's important to note this distinction from conventional cancer treatments.

Integrative medicine is another common term in this discussion. This is a medical approach that combines the rigor of modern science with the wisdom of ancient healing. Its advantages for breast cancer include high-quality scientific evidence for safety and effectiveness; strong patient involvement; low-tech, low-cost approaches; and an overall enhanced sense of patient well-being. "Integrative medicine" is an umbrella term that incorporates complementary therapies, although sometimes the two terms are used interchangeably.

>>> THE 10 BEST QUESTIONS
to Ask Your Doctor About Complementary Therapies
A comprehensive survey by the National Cancer Institute reported that up to 62 percent of American adult cancer patients are using

.org, approximately two-thirds of all people who use complementary medicine don't talk to their doctors about it. Sometimes the doctor lacks formal education in this field or patients are shy about discussing something that seems more about a personal choice, like taking vitamins and herbs. But some herbal supplements can be dangerous and interfere with chemotherapy or other conventional cancer treatments. You may not know this until you talk with your doctor. Ask your doctor to explain your own potential candidacy for complementary therapies rather than give you impersonal CAM statistics.

If your doctor doesn't believe you are a good candidate and you are still interested, ask a follow-up question like, "Do you think I might be able to try a complementary therapy later?" Perhaps after you've gotten through radiation therapy or chemotherapy, you'll be more ready. There may be good reasons for your doctor's current hesitation.

2. Which complementary therapy do you recommend to help me with the physical symptoms from my surgery, chemotherapy, or radiation? Please explain your rationale.

In general, complementary medicine is divided into two classes of therapies, passive and active. A **passive therapy** is one where you let someone do something to you, such as getting a massage or having acupuncture done. An **active therapy** is one where you are the main actor, like taking a yoga class or praying.

THE 10 BEST QUESTIONS TO ASK TO AVOID "CAM SCAMS":

1. **Who's behind this claim or alternative therapy?**

   Any Web site or company offering medical therapies should make it easy to learn who is responsible and what their medical credentials are. Even if someone has initials after his name, question where he works, his training, search his name in Google, and expect to see a list of his publications in professional medical journals. As Quackwatch's Dr. Stephen Barrett warns, "Don't let desperation cloud your judgment."

2. **Are the people offering the alternative therapies also the same people who are selling them?**

   The funding sources behind this Web site should be clearly explained. Information from a neutral or disinterested third party is usually more reliable than information from someone who benefits personally from product sales.

3. **Does this therapy offer a cure, remission, or healing?**

   Alternative therapies include high-dose vitamin supplements, macrobiotic diets, herbal remedies, gadgets, and dietary practices like detoxification. Not all are bad for you or bogus, but the ones that are, such as the drug laetrile, are potentially harmful. Avoid Web sites with flowery medical jargon, claims to cure all cancer (impossible), and multiple ads on the Web site, especially ones that offer money-back guarantees or free trial supplements.

4. **Does the Web site or company have a seal of credibility?**

   If the Web site or company does not have an approval or accreditation seal, that doesn't automatically make it a bogus organization. Check with Health on the Net Foundation (www.hon.ch/) and the URAC (formerly the Utilization Review Accreditation Commission) at www.urac.org to verify seals as one measure of quality.

5. **Is this alternative therapy offered as a "miracle" cure for cancer?**

   Look out for phrases like "scientific breakthrough," "miraculous cure," "secret ingredient," or "ancient remedy." Don't believe claims that say they are credible because they have endured for decades or centuries or have many "testimonials" claiming phenomenal success rates.

...blogs. Be wary of listings that are old or stopped being updated more than a year ago.

8. **Does this alternative therapy or company claim to have exclusive rights to the treatments offered?**

Real cancer treatments are widely available and have been used by hundreds or thousands of cancer patients. Fake cancer treatments are available from only one doctor, clinic, or Web site. It doesn't make sense there would be a monopoly on new products or treatments as good as these claim to be.

9. **Has any conventional medical organization endorsed this product or treatment?**

Endorsements by trusted names in medical science and oncology are a good sign. In contrast, cancer scammers emphasize that others — usually highly respected doctors or cancer centers or "the establishment" — are trying to suppress the distribution of their products.

10. **Is personal information or money requested up front?**

Avoid Web sites that won't give you factual information about their products until you've created an account with them, revealing your name, e-mail address, credit card number, or other personal details. Other red flags include requests for money up front or the seller offering a perpetual discount.

The Magic Question

If a medical breakthrough really had occurred in the treatment of cancer, would the news be announced first in an ad?

The credit for this commonsense question belongs to the Federal Trade Commission, the federal government's watchdog organization. The con artists' claim of "exclusive rights" is the ultimate tip-off that this is a bogus treatment.

Another useful way of understanding the highly diverse field of complementary medicine is by grouping it into categories. The three major categories and examples of complementary therapies are:

- **Touch therapy.** Holistic massages, hands-on healing techniques, Reiki, etc.
- **Mind-body therapy.** Prayer, meditation, music therapy, hypnosis, tai chi, etc.
- **Manipulative and body-based practices.** Acupressure, acupuncture, massage, yoga, etc.

This question focuses on helping your physical symptoms from the cancer or treatments, especially pain management and side effects like nausea. Both active and passive therapies can help to lessen pain, ease tightness across a surgical scar, alleviate nausea, or help to manage lymphedema.

3. Which complementary therapy do you recommend to help me with the emotional or psychological issues about having cancer? Please explain your rationale.

The active and passive therapies listed above can help with psychological or emotional distress. The goal of complementary medicine is to balance the whole person—physically, mentally, and emotionally—while standard cancer treatments (chemo, etc.) are doing their job.

This question may be more difficult to discuss with your doctor, but asking the Best Question 2 above is a good warm-up. Now you've already opened the door for a good discussion that will result in an individualized treatment plan of complementary therapies just for you. Again, make sure you understand why your doctor has recommended this therapy and how long you should continue it.

can lower their heartbeat at will. The relatively recent interest in complementary medicine within the medical community means there aren't as many evidence-based studies as with most other cancer treatments. The key to the answer to this question is to hear the good news (we hope) about your future improvements balanced with a shot of reality on the therapy's potential limitations.

5. Are there any side effects or potential dangers for me if I use these complementary therapies?

There is a wide range of possible side effects across the very diverse spectrum of complementary medicine. Regardless of the therapy, you want to be sure it's safe and effective before you start.

There are virtually no side effects for therapies such as massages, praying, and visualization. Some therapies, including acupuncture, yoga, Pilates, and other exercise programs, have slight risks. Ask your doctor if there are treatment standards or clinical trial results for the therapies you are considering. Discuss with her your prior physical and mental health, along with your current conventional treatment progress as part of this discussion.

6. In your opinion, do the known benefits outweigh the risks for these therapies?

If the answer is no, explore your doctor's rationale.

7. Are there any complementary therapies that I should totally avoid because they will interfere with my other treatments?

As you discuss this question with your doctor, he may wander into a discussion of alternative medicine, too. That's OK, because you need your doctor's wisdom on this, and there is some fuzziness between the two terms. Keep in mind that the difference is that alternative medicine *replaces* conventional cancer treatments, while complementary medicine *adds* to it.

8. Should I let you know before starting a complementary therapy?

This question serves to give you an official stamp of approval on your complementary medicine treatment plan. Also find out your doctor's wishes about staying informed during the duration of your complementary medicine regime. You might not want to report every yoga class to your doctor, but give her the option of stating her preferred protocol.

9. What's the best way to find a certified CAM practitioner or learn more about complementary therapies?

Once you and your doctor together have developed a plan for your complementary therapies, you'll need to find a well-qualified person to help you. If you are choosing a hands-on therapist, such as for massage or acupuncture, this therapist should be licensed by a credible institution. Look up their training institute on the Internet to make sure it's legit. Ask if they belong to a national association in their field, like the American Massage Therapy Association (www .amtamassage.org). Ask how many years total experience they have and how many breast cancer patients they have previously worked with. Shop around if needed.

Interview the practitioner in advance and make sure you feel

or only offer partial coverage. If your doctor, the office staff, or a social worker can't help you with this question, check directly with your insurance carrier for the fine print for any complementary medicine that has a fee associated with it.

> *The bottom line is to be smart and never ever consider using a complementary therapy instead of mainstream care.*
>
> —BARRIE CASSILETH, PH.D., CHIEF OF THE INTEGRATIVE MEDICINE DEPARTMENT, MEMORIAL SLOAN-KETTERING CANCER CENTER

❯ The Magic Question

What's the latest reading you've done on complementary medicine for breast cancer?

This question will help you understand your doctor's own personal interest and knowledge about complementary therapies. Depending on his answer, you'll have a better idea of how much you can rely on him as an information source and a cheerleader for your new yoga class or walking program.

The reality is that CAM is hot. There are ongoing clinical trials looking at issues such as organ toxicity from certain supplements and the benefits of regular exercise like twenty minutes of brisk walking every day. A lot of complementary medicine isn't rocket science but just down-to-earth strategies for a healthier lifestyle and a preventive-care mindset. Your doctor will be somewhere along a continuum of involvement with complementary medicine. From a patient's perspective, it makes good sense to understand your doctor's personal biases and comfort level with this type of cancer therapy.

CONCLUSION

"Complementary therapies do work and keep patients strong to help them get through the therapy. They are very important," says Dr. Barrie Cassileth. She concludes, "The single most important thing for someone interested in complementary medicine is to go for gold standard care in breast cancer. The reason is that with any kind of cancer you have only one shot, and that's the first one." Asking the right questions will help you and your doctor to define the gold standard for you.

THE 10 BEST RESOURCES

American Cancer Society. "Overview: Breast Cancer: Complementary and Alternative Therapies." www.cancer.org/docroot/CRI/content/CRI_2_2_4X_Complementary_and_alternative_therapies_5.asp?sitearea=.

Barrett, Stephen, and Victor Herbert. "Twenty-five Ways to Spot Quacks and Vitamin Pushers." www.quackwatch.com/01QuackeryRelatedTopics/spotquack.html.

Cohen, Isaac, Debu Tripathy, and Mary Tagliaferri. *Breast Cancer: Beyond Convention: The World's Foremost Authorities on Complementary and Alternative Medicine Offer Advice on Healing.* New York: Atria, 2002.

Federal Trade Commission. "FTC Consumer Alert: Virtual 'Treatments' Can Be Real-World Deceptions." www.ftc.gov/bcp/conline/pubs/alerts/mrclalrt.shtm.

Horner, Christine. *Waking the Warrior Goddess: Dr. Christine Horner's Program to Protect Against and Fight Breast Cancer,* revised ed. Laguna Beach, CA: Basic Health Publications, 2007.

Memorial Sloan-Kettering Cancer C...

...ncer.gov/cancer
...ormation/internet.

National Center for Complementary and Alternative Medicine. "Health Information." nccam.nih.gov/.

Weil, Andrew. *Health and Healing: The Philosophy of Integrative Medicine and Optimum Health,* revised ed. Boston: Houghton Mifflin, 2004.

A growing number of women who have a cancerous breast removed choose to have reconstructive surgery. Many women want to feel less self-conscious about their appearance and more confident about their sexuality. It's also a way to avoid a daily reminder about having breast cancer.

Although nothing can replace or duplicate a breast lost to cancer surgery, breast reconstruction by a plastic surgeon can help to restore the look and feel of the missing breast after a mastectomy. This is an elective surgery. There are no right or wrong answers. If you are thinking about having a breast reconstruction, discuss your interest as soon as possible with your oncologist or surgeon and before you have any other surgery. The timing for reconstructive surgery and the specifics for each case differ, and you need to discuss your options with your doctor. Alex Keller, M.D., a board-certified plastic surgeon in New York City, says, "The best reconstructions are done at the same time as the mastectomy. Women need to think seriously about this as opposed to having a delayed surgery. This is not their only opportunity for a reconstruction, but it is the best time."

It is very important that you ask these questions of your surgeon or oncologist before having breast reconstruction. If you don't understand an answer, ask the doctor to explain it. You'll be on the road to making a well-informed decision. Breast reconstruction and even mastectomy are not emergencies. It is more important for you

> *Think of reconstruction as the "good cards." You've been dealt some lousy cards, but reconstruction surgery is a good card.*
> —DR. GREGORY O. DICK, BOARD-CERTIFIED PLASTIC SURGEON

to make the right decision based on the correct information instead of acting too quickly, before you know all the facts and all your options. You may also want to get a second opinion before making your final decision.

>>> THE 10 BEST QUESTIONS
About Breast Reconstruction Surgery

1. Am I a good candidate for reconstructive surgery? Why or why not?

This is a question to ask at least two people—your oncologist or surgeon and yourself.

Breast reconstruction is a highly individualized decision. Women have widely differing outlooks about the importance of restoring the appearance of their breasts and their degree of emotional attachment to their breasts.

For some women, it's very important, says Rockville, Maryland, plastic surgeon Dr. Gregory O. Dick. "Some women want to start reconstruction because they feel it's a way of getting past their diagnosis." But Dr. Dick also notes the importance of making a clear-headed decision: "Keep in mind that there's really no surgery that will erase the memory of the trauma that you're going through."

Reconstructive surgeons have made enormous strides in what they can do, including being able to rebuild nipples and give you a choice of reconstruction procedures. But not all women are candidates for reconstruction. Ask your doctor to explain her rationale along with her answer to this question. Patients who had been radiated before their reconstruction surgery in general are not good

The most common reconstruction technique is the **breast implant.** Implants use artificial material, either silicone gel or saline, in a leak-proof shell that surgically replaces removed breast tissue. The second type of reconstructive surgery is called a **flap surgery** because it uses a tissue flap taken from your own body to replace the removed breast. Tissue from your tummy, back, or buttocks is used to reconstruct your breast. The two most common tissue flap procedures are the **TRAM flap** (transverse rectus abdominis myocutaneous flap), which uses tissue from the lower tummy area; and the **latissimus dorsi flap,** which uses tissue from the upper back.

There are two types of TRAM flaps, the **pedicle flap** and the **free flap,** which differ in how much tissue is moved around. A newer version of the flap–tummy tuck method is called **DIEP reconstruction** (deep inferior epigastric perforator reconstruction), which uses the same fatty tissue from the tummy but leaves your abdominal muscles intact. TRAM flaps are the most common procedure involving natural tissues, but DIEP surgeries are growing in popularity.

Another surgery to consider later is the reconstruction of a nipple for the new breast. After your initial surgery of either a tissue transfer or implant, you may have further surgery to make a nipple and areola (the dark area around your nipple). Using a natural tissue graft from your body, the surgeon creates a small mound to resemble a nipple and then tattoos the skin around the new nipple to create an areola. This surgery is less complicated and can be done on an outpatient basis usually about three to four months after the mastectomy.

Ask if a plastic surgeon can observe your mastectomy. A compassionate and dedicated plastic surgeon may be willing to do this. Ask about skin-sparing mastectomy techniques that will keep more of your natural skin to cover an artificial implant or tissue flap during reconstruction surgery.

3. What are the advantages for each type of reconstructive surgery in my case?

The advantages of a breast implant include its feeling like a natural breast (silicone mimics a natural breast better than saline), flexible sizes, the relative ease of inserting and removing it, thus less recovery time and less cost compared to a more extensive flap surgery described below. (Keep in mind that your insurance may pay for your breast reconstruction, so cost may not matter to you.) If you have an implant inserted at the same time as your mastectomy, you may not need extra hospital time.

The key advantage for any of the flap surgeries is a more natural-looking breast made from your own body tissue. You can skip worrying about implant leakage or future replacements of the saline or silicone gel packs. There are several other flap surgeries with variations in where the tissue is taken from and how the blood vessels are surgically treated. If tissue is removed from your abdomen, you'll get a flat tummy as a nice bonus!

4. What are the risks and safety issues for each type of reconstructive surgery?

As more reconstructive operations are performed, surgical techniques and implants have improved. There are now far fewer complications than just five years ago. However, breast reconstruction is still a major surgery.

tected by:

- What type of breast reconstructive surgery you have chosen
- The timing of your reconstructive surgery (immediate or later)
- Whether or not any lymph nodes were removed during your mastectomy
- How well you take care of yourself before and after surgery

For breast implants, the disadvantages include the hazard of a rupture. This is especially true for silicone implants, because a silicone leak is more likely to be slow and undetected as it seeps into your surrounding tissues. There have been inconclusive studies in the past that have examined the safety of silicone implants. The common wisdom in the medical community these days is that silicone is safe. Ask your doctor about the latest studies and her opinions on this issue. You can also expect pain, swelling, bruising, and tenderness that will last a number of weeks. Your surgeon may need to use a balloon expander to stretch your skin enough to make it ready for a permanent implant.

Health risks for both kinds of breast implants include a hardening of surrounding tissues, infections, pain, and nerve damage. Also be aware that breast implants don't last forever. You'll need to have the implant replaced at some point, which will involve an additional surgery. "Something man-made won't last a lifetime, so the likelihood of going back for a future surgery for implant-related problems is something patients must carry with them," says plastic surgeon Dr. Alex Keller. He adds, "The patient with one implant-related problem might have it replaced but the patient who has had two or more implant-related problems is thinking, What else is there?"

For flap surgeries, the disadvantages include a longer recovery time (six to eight weeks) and greater risks from infections and tissue death resulting from this more invasive surgery. You'll have two surgical sites to protect and heal (your breast and tummy or buttocks), and there can be large scars. Women with a low percentage of body fat may not have enough to spare for flap surgery and therefore won't be good candidates.

Perhaps most importantly, because flap procedures are far more complicated surgeries than implants, you'll need an especially skillful surgeon who is highly experienced and trained in microvascular techniques which involve very small blood vessels. As Dr. Keller points out, "Surgeons need to have done hundreds of DIEP flap procedures before they get really good at it." The DIEP flap procedure is a longer and more complex surgery, which increases the risks of complications during the operation, but patients are likely to recover faster and have more favorable results long term (i.e., intact abdominal muscles) than with the TRAM flap.

5. What will my breast look like and feel like after the surgery?

Your reconstructed breast will not look or feel exactly the same as your natural breast. It may look flatter or more youthful. The skin over your new breast will feel normal, since it's your own skin, but sensation in the new breast is usually different. It may feel either overly sensitive or numb, sometimes with a tingling for the first few weeks. Breast implants are designed to feel soft and pliable like a natural breast.

Getting both breasts to look perfectly ~~...~~
istic expectation. ~~...~~

~~... to reduce~~, enlarge, or lift it
~~...anced~~ look. You can also wear a partial breast form
(prosthesis) to hide an imperfect match.

6. How many surgeries will I need?

Breast reconstruction often involves more than one operation. Be sure to ask this question regardless of which type of reconstruction you are considering. If you choose implants, as already noted you can count on at least one additional surgery over your lifetime to replace the implant. If you choose a flap procedure, you are actually signing on for two surgeries in one—breast reconstruction and a tummy tuck. A tummy tuck might sound tempting, but keep in mind that it's still another surgery that you'll have to recover from. Most women need to have two or three operations to get a good match with the opposite breast. After the initial surgery, you may need further operations to reduce scars and perhaps liposuction to refine the shape of the reconstructed breast. Both Dr. Dick and Dr. Keller concur that a high percentage of their patients (between 75 and 90 percent) eventually decide to have a nipple reconstruction. Many women wait until later for this procedure.

7. What will happen if I'm not happy with the results?

Your expectations—and how realistic you are—set the stage for how likely you are to be pleased with the results of your breast reconstruction surgery. Be sure to discuss your expectations and this question with your surgeon before you decide to have the surgery.

Listen to your plastic surgeon's answer to this question as a window into understanding her philosophy on patient-centered care. For example, Dr. Dick noted how important it is to him that his patients feel free to contact him. He says, "I see myself as a navigator who can help you." Likewise, Dr. Keller commented, "Patients appreciate up-front honesty. It's an operation. Of course there are going to be complications."

Also think to ask this question from the perspective of your long-term happiness. For example, two factors that might affect the appearance of your reconstructed breast over time are your aging body and a substantial weight loss or gain. Get a clear picture of factors that could later affect your satisfaction.

8. When should I plan for this reconstructive surgery, and how does scheduling it fit into my total treatment plan?

Don't feel rushed into deciding on reconstructive surgery. "There are very few patients that have cancer so advanced they can't have breast reconstruction done at the time of the initial mastectomy," says Dr. Keller. Knowing how and when your reconstructive surgery fits into your total treatment plan will give you an increased sense of control during this tough time and a certain peace of mind.

If postmastectomy radiation therapy is planned, it can cause complications with either breast implants or tissue flap procedures. Radiation therapy may change the skin's texture, cosmetic appearance, or cause the reconstructed breast to shrink. Therefore, most surgeons prefer to postpone breast reconstruction until after radiation therapy is completed.

...recurrence of breast cancer. It should not cause problems with further chemotherapy or radiation treatment if cancer does recur. If you are considering either an implant or tissue flap procedure, you need to know that reconstruction rarely, if ever, hides a return of breast cancer on a mammogram. Studies support continued mammograms of tissue flap breast reconstructions. Cancer can recur in the skin or any remaining breast tissue at the breast reconstruction site. If you have a tissue flap reconstruction, you may need to continue mammograms on both breasts. Every case of breast cancer is different. Be sure to ask your oncologist and surgeon about any concerns you should have based on your own diagnosis, tumor type, and stage.

10. What can I expect during recovery?

Your surgeon's answer will vary greatly depending on what type of surgery you are having, when (with the mastectomy or later), and your current general health. Recovery time may increase if you have other major health problems, such as diabetes or heart disease.

Your ability to get back to work and your daily routine will depend on how strenuous your job and what your daily routines are. For example, if you have a TRAM flap procedure and have young children, your surgeon will advise you to avoid lifting or carrying them for a longer time than if you had had a simpler breast implant. The second site (abdomen, back, or buttock) for the tissue flap surgery requires more healing time than implants. Ask about possible postsurgical complications such as lymphedema (swelling in your arm), wound care, pain, and how often you'll need follow-up office exams.

Also ask if you will need at-home care, rehabilitation services, or physical therapy as part of your immediate recovery. If so, you'll need to make these arrangements before entering the hospital. You should be up and around in six to eight weeks for a flap procedure, less time for implants. Realistically, it may take up to two years for your incisions to heal fully and the scars to fade. Realize that the scars will never go away completely.

❯ The Magic Question

What is your conversion rate from DIEP flap surgeries to TRAM flap surgeries?

If you are considering having a DIEP tissue flap surgery or another of the more complex flap reconstructive surgeries, it's really important not to have a rookie surgeon. Dr. Keller, who specializes in these surgeries, says this is the Magic Question to ask about flaps. "Most plastic surgeons know how to do an implant, but significantly fewer plastic surgeons know how to do a flap procedure," he says.

Because of the surgical skill involved in a DIEP flap surgery, some less experienced surgeons end up converting the surgery to a TRAM during the operation. The patient doesn't know this until she wakes up. You want to know before you go under the knife how often this surgeon actually does the surgery he says he is going to do. You are looking for patterns of problems or inexperience.

CONCLUSION

Still not sure what to do? Here's the bottom line from Dr. Gregory Dick. He believes that if you are really unsure about whether or not you want reconstructive surgery it's h---

RESOURCES

American Cancer Society. "Breast Reconstruction After Mastectomy." www.cancer.org/docroot/CRI/content/CRI_2_6X_Breast_Reconstruction _After_Mastectomy_5.asp.

American Society of Plastic Surgeons. "Breast Reconstruction." www .plasticsurgery.org/patients_consumers/procedures/BreastReconstruction .cfm.

Baker, Sherry. "Making the Choice: What You Need to Know about Breast Reconstruction." *MAMM Magazine*, September–October 2005. www .mamm.com.

Berger, Karen, and John Bostwick. *A Woman's Decision: Breast Care, Treatment & Reconstruction*, 3rd ed. New York: St. Martin's Griffin, 1998.

BreastImplantSafety.org. "Breast Reconstruction." www.breastimplant safety.org/BreastReconstruction/index.php.

Chesser, Carla. *Laughing through the Tears of Breast Cancer: My Personal Metamorphosis*. Victoria, British Columbia: Trafford Publishing, 2006.

Food and Drug Administration. "Breast Implants Home Page." www.fda .gov/cdrh/breastimplants/.

Love, Susan, Karen Lindsey, and Marcia Williams. "Reconstruction and Prosthesis: Making a Decision," in *Dr. Susan Love's Breast Book*, 4th ed. Cambridge: Da Capo Press, 2005.

National Cancer Institute. "Fact Sheet: National Cancer Institute Breast Implant Study." www.cancer.gov/cancertopics/factsheet/siliconefactsheet.

Steligo, Kathy. *The Breast Reconstruction Guidebook*, 2nd ed. San Carlos, CA: Carlo Press, 2005.

This section of the book helps you deal with the practical realities of your need for emotional, financial, and social well-being following your diagnosis of breast cancer. By using the following 10 Best Questions lists, you'll be much more likely to understand and conquer your fears and the uncertainties about the other aspects of your personal life that have been affected by your diagnosis.

You can go a long way toward assessing your emotional stability and financial health by asking yourself the 10 Best Questions in these chapters. There are also chapters in this section to guide you during the most difficult conversations you are likely to have with the people closest to you—your partner (including conversations about sex and intimacy), other loved ones, and your children. Your loved ones and friends ultimately become breast cancer survivors, too. The chapter on support groups will help you choose new friends and join the "sisterhood" wisely. The last chapter on the 10 Worst Questions is partly just for fun and also a gentle reminder that sometimes even well-intentioned people just don't know what to ask you.

The Question Doctor sincerely hopes this information will serve as your companion and be a guiding force as you redefine the relationships in your life and strive to make peace with your emotional and financial needs.

Australian pop singer and actress,

on being diagnosed with breast cancer

A diagnosis of breast cancer is not only life threatening but also emotionally transformative. Cancer can be a powerful wake-up call for change and a catalyst for you to stop and examine your emotions, your coping skills, your relationships, and yourself.

Most women's initial reactions to their diagnosis include feeling overwhelmed, shocked, angry, scared silly, confused, and oftentimes very alone.

Typically the patient, her loved ones, and her medical team all go into hyperdrive to combat the physical effects of the disease. Treatment plans, side effects, and hair loss become your standard topics at the dinner table. All attention zooms in on making you healthy again.

But you also need to ask yourself, What about my emotional life? Oncologist Dr. Marisa C. Weiss shares her insights: "You need to look out for your emotional health because the mind is the most powerful organ that you have. If there's a disconnection between the emotions and the physical, or you are ignoring your emotional life or don't understand confusing feelings, your relationships become jarred and disconnected. Everything you're doing to get well will become much more difficult."

These Best Questions have no right or wrong answers—only

JOURNALING

When they are first diagnosed, some women start a journal of everything that is happening to them—what the doctor says, when and what the treatments are, and what they learned from Web sites or books about breast cancer. Others prefer to keep a more reflective personal journal of how they are feeling, their relationships with loved ones, spiritual thoughts or prayers, hopes, dreams, and reasons for gratitude.

If you like this idea, find your own way of journaling. Try to write something every day. It's a wonderful outlet for making sense of your emotions and creating a record of valuable information about your breast cancer. Just let your anger, frustration, and uncertainties flow onto the page without self-criticism or editing.

As a written response to your daily life, your journal can identify changes or patterns in your moods and emotions, stress levels, energy levels, and work productivity. This insight can be psychologically and physically uplifting. Journaling shouldn't feel like a chore. Take a time out when you need to or make a change from writing by dedicating a page to a quick sketch, a meaningful quote, or a photograph. Feel free to customize your journal with the things that best tell your own story.

Beverly Kirkhart, breast cancer survivor and co-author of *Chicken Soup for the Surviving Soul: 101 Healing Stories About Those Who Have Survived Cancer,* says, "I believe in using the tool of journaling. I approached my breast cancer that way. When my feelings popped up I could address them in my journal."

degrees of emotional honesty or dishonesty with yourself. Share these questions and your responses with others only if you want to. Breast cancer survivors and experts all agree that it does get better with time. Keep these Best Questions close by for when you need them along the way.

>>>THE 10 BEST QUEST...

...angry, hurt, shocked, or in denial as you read this.

To help yourself understand and get beyond your current negative feelings, think back to what was going on in your emotional life on that day you first heard "breast cancer." What was going on for you emotionally, socially, in your love relationships, relationships with family members, friends, and coworkers? Maybe you had an argument with your mother or teenager or were in the midst of watching your marriage slowly dissolve. Or perhaps life was good. You were planning a romantic getaway cruise and have a new grandbaby who looks like you. Whatever was going on—both the good stuff and the bad stuff—all becomes amplified and magnified after a cancer diagnosis.

This "emotional audit" will help you keep the past (prediagnosis) in its proper perspective. Most women can remember vividly how they felt when they were first told they had breast cancer. Whatever your initial feelings, you will probably go on to experience many different emotions during your cancer journey. This is the starting point—square one—for the rest of the following Best Questions.

2. What coping strategies have been most successful for me in the past?

This Best Question was suggested by Patricia Ganz, M.D., director of cancer prevention and control research at UCLA's Jonsson Comprehensive Cancer Center. Dr. Ganz has spent twenty years researching the emotional impact of breast cancer, and she says, "People bring to bear whatever coping strategies they had before. 'Approach-oriented coping,' trying to acknowledge what the problem is, can be effective for women with breast cancer."

Use this Best Question to hang on to whatever is the best part of you from the past crises in your life. Think back to the most dramatic past tragedies that have touched you. What did you do well to handle those situations? What do you wish you had done better? What were your "lessons learned" from those experiences?

3. How do I feel about my physical changes and body image?

Our society places a great emphasis on a woman's breasts. Breasts are equated to a woman's sexuality, attractiveness, desirability, and femininity. Because of these attitudes, breast cancer can deeply undermine your self-image and erode your self-confidence in intimate relationships.

All breast cancer patients have their own feelings about their breasts and what they have meant to them in their lives—erogenous zones, breastfeeding, or memories of past favorite bikinis. Looking and feeling good is important to women dealing with unfun stuff like surgeries, side effects, and unpredictable relationships. Regardless of whether you've had a lumpectomy, mastectomy, double mastectomy, or no surgery, the psychological effects on your sense of self-worth and body image are still very real.

"What helped me to face the mastectomy were two things I heard from both my friends and my oncologist—'Boobs are overrated' and 'It's to save your life.' I found myself saying those two things over and over again when I began to think I couldn't face another step," said Sandra, forty-three, in Lansing, Michigan.

"Before I went for chemotherapy, I would dress up: full makeup, smart clothes, the works. It was a bit of a false face, but it did make me feel like less of

...more than you may realize at first. It's only natural to be thinking about yourself right now. As social worker and experienced counselor Pat Spicer at CancerCare observes, "Women are often caught up in their own feelings and never think about what the other person is going through."

But others' reactions can greatly impact your own emotional well-being. For example, if your beloved brother is freaking out and terribly fearful for you, it's only human nature that you'll absorb and reflect back some of his fear, too. Perhaps your partner just doesn't know what to do, so he or she is treating you like you are made out of glass, totally fragile and breakable at any minute. First, you have to avoid the trap of thinking like that yourself. The last thing you want right now is to feel helpless. Most women complain about feeling out of control, and sometimes well-intentioned partners contribute to this feeling. Second, you've got to find a gentle way to ask your well-intentioned partner to stop so there are no hurt feelings or bitterness.

In another scenario, you run into an occasional friend at the local grocery store and tell her about your breast cancer—and she starts sobbing hysterically. Now you've got to comfort her, instead of the other way around. Unfortunately, this happens all too often, and it can wear you down, especially when it is combined with all the other stress and uncertainty in your life right now.

It's also possible that you are assuming a lot of reactions that aren't necessarily so. Maybe you think your work colleagues are annoyed with you or feel like you're not pulling your weight on the job these days because of your time off for appointments and treatments. It could be that this is the furthest thing from their minds.

If you ask yourself this Best Question before talking with others about their reactions to your cancer, it will help you to clarify what's really going on. Be kind to yourself and your loved ones. And be aware that you may have to take care of some of them just when you need their help the most. Dr. Robert Granet, in his book *Surviving Cancer Emotionally: Learning How to Heal*, calls loved ones "second-order patients" who need care, too.

5. Where can I get help? Who are my best resources for support?

Don't be afraid to ask for help. It doesn't mean you are helpless or weak. Far from it. Asking for help means conserving your energy to get well. You don't have to face your breast cancer alone.

There are many sources for emotional help and many sets of listening ears when you need them (besides your pet dog or cat). These include your partner, family members, friends, local support groups, online support communities, social workers, your doctors, oncology nurses, nurse navigators, clergy or other religious leaders, community leaders, and professional therapists and psychiatrists.

Some women team up with "cancer buddies," either with a friend who has survived breast cancer or from a referral offered by various local or national services that provide a face-to-face comrade or a virtual pal. Just having someone who cares and listens to you can make a world of difference in your emotional well-being during the healing process.

6. What am I denying or avoiding about my diagnosis? (Stage 1)

Let's face it. Most of us go through life without really believing we are going to die someday. Our own death seems like an abstract

...nge of a job promotion can trigger grief. She also emphasized that you can slip back into stage 2 after you've moved into stage 3 or even skip a stage entirely. Getting stuck at a stage is a common problem and could be the source of much of your anguish. The five stages are:

1. **Denial and shock.** The initial stage: "Cancer can't be happening to me."
2. **Anger.** "Why me? This isn't fair. I don't deserve cancer."
3. **Bargaining.** "Just let me live to see my grandchildren."
4. **Depression.** "I'm so sad, why bother with anything?"
5. **Acceptance.** "I'm going to be OK and make it through."

Best Questions 6 through 10 in this chapter use Dr. Kübler-Ross's stages as a framework to help you get in touch with your deepest emotional responses to having breast cancer. This is not to imply that you are going to die, but rather to help you understand your emotions — and your grief — based on Dr. Kübler-Ross's extensive research.

event off in the distant future. After a diagnosis of breast cancer, this abstraction is often a sudden and harsh reality. The lid on our illusions has been ripped off.

The key way people have of coping with such news is shock and denial. That's why people's initial reactions at first diagnosis are almost universally being overwhelmed and shocked and denying the news. By letting the new information dribble in slowly, in pieces, and over time instead of instantaneously, this defense mechanism prevents the brain from shutting down entirely.

Being in shock is why most women never hear anything their doctors say beyond "You've got breast cancer." Your whole soul aches to return to your normal life before those words. As author and former NBC correspondent Betty Rollin advises, based on her own experience with breast cancer, "You can't overload your emotional state before you are ready."

Many medical doctors have a strictly clinical approach to treating cancer which can also contribute to your getting stuck at the denial stage. As UCLA's Dr. Patricia Ganz explains, "The average doctor, even a very skilled physician, is not very tuned in to patients' psychosocial needs. If your doctor is not meeting your psychosocial needs, ask for help. If you aren't sleeping, for example, ask for medications or counseling that will help you."

What matters the most is how well you deal with your diagnosis after the initial shock has worn off. Dr. Ganz and other experts emphasize the importance of moving on from this stage. She says, "Women who avoid dealing with their emotions have more troubles downstream." One effective method is to focus on learning more about your disease, thus empowering yourself with facts, questions, and answers.

7. How can I channel my anger into a positive healing experience? (Stage 2)

Most breast cancer patients feel like their lives have been hijacked by their disease. How could my body betray me like this? How fast can I get my damn breast off and go back to normal?

Nearly everyone goes through the stage of anger—anger at themselves, anger at God, anger at those around them, anger at their doctors, and anger at their fate. Sometimes other feelings, like fear, anxiety, worry, or panic are expressed as angry outbursts. Caregivers and loved ones are also often angry with themselves, their family members, or the patient. There's often anger at God because it seems like He is unjustly punishing you, especially if you believe you've lived a fairly

... you find yourself stuck or returning to the anger stage, seek professional counseling or other outside support sources. By all means, don't stay angry forever.

8. What am I bargaining for either consciously or unconsciously? (Stage 3)

Dr. Kübler-Ross describes this stage in her book *On Death and Dying:*

> The bargaining is really an attempt to postpone; it has to include a prize offered "for good behavior," it also sets a self-imposed deadline . . . and an implicit promise the patient will not ask for more if one postponement is granted . . . like children who say, "I will never fight with my sister again" . . . Needless to add, the little boy will fight with his sister again, just like the opera singer will try to perform once more . . . Most bargains are made with God and usually kept a secret.

Reflect for yourself; does this sound familiar? Ultimately, many women find positive outlets for improving their lives and expressing kind and charitable actions. For example, this stage can serve as a launchpad for personal involvement in Breast Cancer Awareness Month activities, volunteering as a support group leader, or making a contribution to a breast cancer foundation.

Dr. Kübler-Ross also discusses the role of fear as a major contributor to a bargaining mindset. Fear is a very powerful emotion and a very common reaction to a diagnosis of breast cancer. But because we can't just say we'll get over our fears, we try to bargain them away or deny their existence. Fear plays a heavy role in your choice of treatments, decisions on surgery, and your general reactions to your diagnosis.

In the book *How Not to Be Afraid of Your Own Life: Opening Your Heart to Confidence, Intimacy, and Joy,* author Susan Piver suggests these tips for a more fearless life: let yourself be afraid, ask for help, put others first, cheer up, relax, stop talking to yourself, bring someone with you, time it, listen to the silence, and learn to meditate.

9. How can I better cope with my feelings of being overly stressed and depressed? (Stage 4)

Advanced oncology nurse Melissa Craft has spent thirty years helping cancer patients cope with their emotions. She says, "Breast cancer patients have an overwhelming sense of isolation. Just because there are millions of survivors of breast cancer doesn't mean you don't feel alone with yours." Common signs of stress include disturbed sleep, fatigue, body aches, pain, anxiety, irritability, tension, and headaches. Depression is frequently caused by feeling too much stress over time.

One key strategy in order to move beyond this stage, which is where many women get stuck during their cancer journeys, is to focus on being better prepared to make the best decisions you possibly can. Arm yourself with as much factual information as you can and as you are able to handle. It's also normal and very common to have trouble taking in and understanding medical information when you are emotionally overwrought.

If you are already feeling defeated and drained, try these techniques to rebound:

- Rest your mind

- Avoid "hard news," like war reports, politics, or murders.

Depression is a common yet often unrecognized source of suffering among women with breast cancer. It is a highly treatable symptom that often accompanies the cancer experience. The signs of depression include frequent feelings of sadness or emptiness, finding little or no pleasure in life, crying spells, having loved ones who comment on your sadness, and feeling worthless or suicidal. Seek professional help to treat your depression if it is interfering with your life, your cancer treatments, or your recovery.

10. What steps can I take to accept my cancer? How can I put to rest any feelings of guilt or blame? (Stage 5)

Acceptance as described by Dr. Kübler-Ross means coming to grips with your fate and tuning the lemons you've been handed (breast cancer) into lemonade (the cloud with a silver lining). She believed that it's the acknowledgment of grief over change or a pending loss (such as a breast removed) that holds the key to living or dying well, with dignity and grace.

Another version of this Best Question is, "How can I treat myself with more compassion?" Acceptance and self-love are very important to helping you overcome the psychological impact that some women experience because they blame themselves for their breast cancer. Suggesting that the patient is somehow to blame is a common phenomenon.

When Jacqueline Kennedy Onassis died in 1994 from non-Hodgkin's lymphoma, a form of cancer, the tabloid headlines screamed, "Did a life of tragedy cause her fatal cancer?" You may find yourself wondering similarly, "Did the stress at work cause my cancer?" "Did my teenage years of eating 2:00 a.m. pizzas, smoking dope, and drinking diet sodas cause my cancer?" Sometimes insensitive or uneducated people blurt out questions like, "Why did you get cancer?" as if you had had a choice or any control.

Many women worry incessantly about what behavior or action caused their cancer. At the present time, we don't know what causes most cancers. You might fear for your other family members, but only a small percentage of cancers are known to be hereditary.

There is nothing taboo about cancer, and it's not contagious. It's not something you "did" to yourself. Tell your friends to throw away their surgical masks when they see you coming. You aren't radioactive (even if you've had radiation therapy), you aren't an alien life form, and you don't have to wear a giant scarlet *C* on your chest like you're some kind of broken-down cancer floozy.

Lose that big scarlet *C* and you're well on your way to passing the "acceptance test" with flying colors.

❯ The Magic Question

How can I feel my best today?

Many breast cancer patients allow their diagnosis, external circumstances, and other people to determine how they feel.

You can take back control of your feelings by asking yourself this Magic Question. Your renewed sense of self-worth and confidence for living is priceless. As Dr. Susan Love, breast cancer guru, says, "Be patient with yourself and with others. Try to remember: Most women don't die of breast cancer, and most do not have to lose their breast."

CONCLUSION

...........y. Anxiety, Fear, and Depression." www.cancer
.org/docroot/MBC/MBC_4x_Anxiety.asp?sitearea=MBC.

American Cancer Society. "Coping with Physical and Emotional Changes."
www.cancer.org/docroot/MBC/MBC_0.asp.

American Cancer Society. "Reach to Recovery Program." www.cancer.org/
docroot/ESN/content/ESN_3_1x_Reach_to_Recovery_5.asp?sitearea=
SHR.

American Psychological Oncology Society. "Organizations and Information for Cancer Patients and Caregivers." www.apos-society.org/survivors/
resources/organizations.aspx.

CancerCare. "Get Help/Cancercare Counseling." www.cancercare.org/
get_help/help_by_diagnosis/diagnosis.php?diagnosis=breast.

Canfield, Jack, Mark Victor Hansen, and Mary Olsen Kelly. *Chicken Soup
for the Breast Cancer Survivor's Soul: Stories to Inspire, Support and Heal*, 2nd
ed. Deerfield Beach, FL: HCI, 2006.

Holland, Jimmie, and Sheldon Lewis. *The Human Side of Cancer: Living
with Hope, Coping with Uncertainty*. New York: Harper Paperbacks, 2001.

National Cancer Institute. "Anxiety Disorder (PDQ)." www.cancer.gov/
cancertopics/pdq/supportivecare/anxiety/patient.

National Cancer Institute. "Depression (PDQ)." www.cancer.gov/cancer
topics/pdq/supportivecare/depression/patient.

National Cancer Institute. "Facing Forward: Life After Cancer Treatment." www.cancer.gov/cancertopics/life-after-treatment.

A support group is a number of people who meet together on a regular basis in the presence of a trained group leader (also called a "facilitator") to discuss their experiences, feelings, fears, needs, and questions. There are also moderated and nonmoderated online support groups.

The goal of a support group is to help you restore the self-confidence that your breast cancer has undermined, to redefine your life, to connect with a community of understanding people, and to learn more about breast cancer. (The terms "members" and "participants" are used interchangeably here, but some groups make distinctions between regular and occasional attendees.) There are many advantages to belonging to a support group. These include allowing you to:

- Connect with others who are going through the same thing
- Overcome feelings of isolation, fear, and being overwhelmed
- Get insider information on the best doctors, cancer care centers, books, and Web sites
- Express confusing or frightening emotions in a safe environment
- Feel less helpless and learn where to get more help
- Learn more about breast cancer

- Give loved ones touched by cancer (partner, family, and friends) an outlet, too

As noted by an oncology nurse in Barbara Delinsky's book *Uplift: Secrets from the Sisterhood of Breast Cancer Survivors,* "A breast cancer diagnosis puts you into an exclusive club. You wouldn't choose to join it, but once you do, you find a sisterhood like no other."

>>> THE 10 BEST QUESTIONS
Before Joining a Support Group

1. Who leads the group? What is this person's background, formal training, and experience with breast cancer patients and their families?

The skill and experience level of the group leader can make a night and day difference in how much you enjoy the group and how much you benefit from it. A well-led group will greatly reduce the risk that your support group experience will be negative or hurtful. Poorly run support groups can actually damage a cancer survivor's emotional stability, which is usually under siege anyway from the stress of the diagnosis and treatments.

The group leader sets the meeting's tone, structure, and agenda, as well as controls the group's discussion patterns. It's important that no one member dominate the discussions and equally important that all members feel free to participate if they choose to. This is much easier said than done, and it takes a highly experienced group leader to make the group run smoothly. An excellent facilitator knows how to accommodate changes in the group's size and participant mix, as well as how to draw all people equally into the conversations, regardless of the topic or members' personalities.

The key role of the group leader is to provide support, structure,

GILDA'S CLUB WORLDWIDE

... clinic for over twenty-five years.

Joanna Bull shared her insights on group leaders during an interview with this author: "In general, it's preferable to have a trained facilitator rather than a volunteer who has had breast cancer because the group is dealing with the extremely complex and profound issues of living and dying. At Gilda's Club we 'untrain' our facilitators. We want them to use their professional skills but not be seen as the experts with all the answers. The real experts are the members of the group with the experience of living with cancer. It takes a humble facilitator to do this, but it is actually quite freeing as time goes on."

and security for the members, not to tell her own cancer stories or to voice personal opinions. Ask if the facilitator is a licensed social worker, marriage counselor, or psychotherapist with substantive training and/or experience in managing group dynamics to help clarify this person's expertise.

According to social worker and support group veteran Pat Spicer, "Look for a support group led by a professional facilitator, such as an oncology nurse or an oncology social worker or a pastoral counselor. Insist that the facilitator have a background in oncology. The issues for an oncology patient are very different than heart patients, for example."

Also be on the lookout for a burned-out facilitator, someone who might be experienced but who feels personally worn out from absorbing so much emotional pain over an extended time. The worst group leader is someone who has a lot of personal problems

THE QUESTION DOCTOR SAYS:

The best trained and most experienced group leaders understand that not everyone wants the details of their lives and breast cancer blabbed all around town. Find out how the group leader and members deal with confidentiality issues.

herself and therefore can't act like a neutral sounding board, a role essential to free-flowing sharing.

2. What does the group talk about?

What happens in most support groups is a sharing of commonalities, fears, and feelings. Some groups also offer educational segments or guest speakers, but most groups are forums for participants to talk openly about what's happening with them personally as they move through their cancer journeys.

A key component of support group discussions should be community building. This means that the group leader and participants are creating a warm atmosphere where all comments are welcomed without judgment or criticism and can be voiced without restraint.

If you aren't sure about what the group talks about in advance, give it a try for several sessions and see if the group's discussion topics and focus match your own needs. If not, you might consider try-

People with a great deal of experience with support groups — both as cancer patients and group leaders — caution against joining an overly optimistic group. In these groups, cancer patients are expected to be constantly positive, the conversations always upbeat, and smiles all around. Our society's standard of positive thinking forces some to deny the inherent sadness within a cancer diagnosis. Look for a group that doesn't dwell on grief and sadness but also doesn't force false cheerfulness from its participants.

ing at least one ~~~

..~~~, patients with metastatic disease, and groups consisting of mixed stages of breast cancer.

The same grouping holds true for prostate cancer and other types of cancer as well. Sometimes group members have nothing in common but cancer; other times the members are nearly homogenous in their ages, cancer types and stages, and their emotional needs. As Claudia Lee, a breast cancer center consultant in Hudson, New York, says, "A support group for newly diagnosed women is very different than a support group for women who have recurred."

4. Are the participants either patients or family members or both in a mixed group?

The general consensus among support group experts is that separate support groups for patients and for family members/friends work best. "If you and he [your partner] are in the same group, there'll be issues that you won't feel comfortable bringing up," points out Joanna Bull.

There may be some circumstances where you may want to be with your partner, family, or friends, but in general breast cancer patients have their own needs best met by other breast cancer patients, even more than by their closest loved ones. Pat Spicer comments, "For women who are dealing with their breast cancer diagnosis, it's almost like they have learned another language. Now they need to speak to others in that new language."

Likewise, loved ones have unique needs as caregivers and common issues to share among themselves that may not be fully appreciated by even the most empathetic cancer patients. If you want to address relationship changes or challenges, check into options for couples-only support groups either in your community or online. If you can't find a group in your area, some caregivers say Web sites with support groups have helped them a lot.

5. What is the size and turnover of the group?

The best support groups have at least six members at each session and no more than twenty at a time. If there are fewer than six in attendance, the conversation may lag or become fixated on just one or two dominant personalities. In groups larger than fifteen, women who are naturally shyer may hesitate to open up, and even confident members may never get a turn. In general, an ideal number is about ten, which helps to ensure diversity yet encourages intimacy, comfort, and trust.

Asking about the members' turnover may not be something that occurs to you as you are first joining a support group, but it's an important question. What this question is really getting at is the issue of commitment. For example, if you feel really involved with a support group over the long haul, you may find it disruptive to have a constant stream of newcomers who show up only infrequently or are never seen again. Each time a new member joins,

National Public Radio journalist and breast cancer survivor Susan Stamberg shares her long-term perspective on support groups: "I'm not much of a group person. I do one-on-one interviews that are heard by millions of people. But the one-on-oneness is what's important to me, and I carry that into my private life. At the time of my diagnosis, I was anchoring a daily news program and was something of a public figure. It was important to me to keep my diagnosis private. Later, I had some regrets about having held so much inside. It might have been helpful, even healthier, to share what I was going through with a wider range of people."

time is spent on introductions

...support group members socialize at times beside
the regular group meetings?

This question may not be relevant to you, especially if the group is comprised of members from a large geographical area or is an online group. Or you may care a lot about having the option of continuing budding friendships in settings beyond a drab hospital or community center meeting room.

7. Who is sponsoring the group and why?

Many support groups are sponsored by a local hospital or medical organization. Call your local hospital or ask your oncologist, nurse navigator, or a social worker for suggestions and local meeting schedules.

There are also many choices among national nonprofit organizations. These include the American Cancer Society's Reach to Recovery Program (www.cancer.org) which has a thirty-year history of helping breast cancer patients cope through locally led support groups, online services, and telephone arrangements. Another giant in this field is the Wellness Community (www.thewellnesscommunity.org), with its twenty-five-year track record of helping people with cancer to connect and feel supported. Gilda's Club (www.gildasclub.org) is another example, as well as Y-Me National Breast Cancer Organization (www.y-me.org) and CancerCare (www.cancercare.org).

In general, your best bet is to look for Web sites that end in

".org." This designation signifies that the organization is not-for-profit and has met tax-related criteria to prove it. These support groups are generally free or low cost. However, that doesn't imply that there's necessarily anything shady or less inviting for support groups with ".com" Web site addresses.

8. Where does the group hold its meetings?

For some people who are choosing a face-to-face support group, a hospital setting is fine, more convenient, and perhaps the only choice in their community. But generally, hospitals are less physically comfortable than a more neutral, inviting environment. Hospitals may trigger negative reactions or memories of your prior unpleasant experiences there during appointments or treatments. There are also church-based support groups, ones that meet in restaurants or private homes, and telephone groups with no physically grounded home base.

Gilda's Club and some other national groups focus on providing pleasant, home-like surroundings to help spark patients' and caregivers' personal connections and soothe their jarred emotions. If location is important to you, choose a group with this in mind. If you prefer an online support group or just don't care about where the meetings are held, then this question won't matter to you.

9. Is there an online component?

Many major organizations, such as the American Cancer Society and Gilda's Club, offer online alternatives to their face-to-face formats. You might like participating in some combination of online activity along with making face-to-face or voice connections. If you are already Internet savvy and enjoy online social networking Web sites such as Facebook and chat rooms, are squeezed for time by a crazy schedule, have limited transportation options, or live in a small community or geographically li...

...tely. Some people choose to attend just during times of change or crisis in their illness or when trying to make decisions.

Closed groups have a consistent group membership. The same people meet for a prescribed period of time and may be organized according to similar diagnosis or cancer stage, by sex, or by the kind of treatments the participants are currently undergoing (chemotherapy, etc.). Sometimes groups are created around specific issues, like certain side effects or types of treatments. Some groups are run by professionals and others by cancer survivors.

In addition to live and online group meetings, there are one-on-one pairings such as mentor-protégé arrangements (experienced patient paired with newcomer), "cancer buddies" (peer pairing), and telephone trees. You may also benefit from talking with a professional counselor, therapist, or psychiatrist. In private sessions with a counselor or therapist, you'll receive maximum attention to your issues as well as the most highly trained advice possible.

Author and patient advocate Marti Ann Schwartz shares her own experiences with a private counselor: "The best thing I ever did was I saw a cancer counselor. She's wonderful and put things into perspective. She knew things that I didn't know and could tell me what happens for other people."

> I needed to be with other women who spoke my same cancer language, who understood that it still isn't over even when your treatments end.
>
> —MARIAH, THIRTY-SEVEN, WASHINGTON, D.C.

❯ The Magic Question

How does the group leader protect the participants' feelings and egos during group discussions?

There is nothing riskier than sharing your most private feelings and revelations in a support group meeting. The most skillful and experienced group leaders understand the need to create a secure and safe discussion environment where you'll feel free to share anything on your mind. Chances are that confidentiality, privacy, and a sense of security during the meetings are all important to you.

One way highly skilled facilitators manage touchy topics is by creating and enforcing ground rules for discussion. These don't have to be complicated or authoritarian. Simple ground rules may include statements posted on the wall like "Everyone's comments are welcome"; "Silence is OK"; "Everyone participates but no one dominates"; "All opinions are OK but no personal attacks"; and "All comments will be confidential and kept inside this room."

Once group members feel secure, they are able to trust the others and really open up. Knowing that the group leader is willing to intervene on your behalf if someone else says something unpleasant or tries to provoke conflict can be very empowering.

CONCLUSION

There are oceans of feelings to process after a diagnosis of breast cancer. Reaching out for help isn't a sign of weakness, but rather shows your strength, self-confidence, and willingness to let others help you. There is a positive connection between asking for help and self-respect.

"A good support group becomes a good community. Support groups are also great resources for educational support, too," says CancerCare's Pat Spicer.

...g. ...root/ESN/esn_3.asp?sitearea=ESN.

American Cancer Society. "Support Groups: General Information." www .cancer.org/docroot/ESN/content/ESN_2_3X_Support_groups_general_ information.asp.

Breastcancer.org. "Support and Community." www.breastcancer.org/ community/index.jsp.

CancerCare. "Online Support Groups." supportgroups.cancercare.org/.

Gilda's Club Worldwide. "Cancer Support for the Whole Family." www .gildasclub.org.

Living Beyond Breast Cancer. "Programs and Services." www.lbbc.org/ programs.asp.

National Breast Cancer Foundation. "Online Discussion." www.national breastcancer.org/mynbcf/discussions.

National Cancer Institute. "Fact Sheet: Cancer Support Groups: Questions and Answers." www.cancer.gov/cancertopics/factsheet/sup port/support-groups.

Susan G. Komen for the Cure. "Find Komen in Your Area." cms.komen .org/komen/Affiliates/index.htm.

Wellness Community. "Find a Wellness Community Near You." www .thewellnesscommunity.org.

—Walter Matthau,
actor

Breast cancer affects not just your health; it also affects your money. But please don't hyperventilate while reading this chapter. Getting a handle on your assets, debts, estate, and having a will doesn't mean you are going to die from breast cancer. It also doesn't mean that you have to do this research alone. If you have a partner or loved one who is itching to volunteer support and is good with numbers, this is a great opportunity to put him or her to work.

Knowing your current financial situation in more detail may actually give you a sense of relief and empowerment. For example, a recent survey found that even in households with an annual income under $100,000, those with financial plans saved twice as much as households without plans. Unlike your cancer, you at least have some control over your finances.

You may not want to spend your energy on financial matters just now. Maybe you basically dislike handling money matters. Whatever your financial status is, think of your diagnosis as a wake-up call to get more financially savvy. Having breast cancer can be expensive in ways you didn't anticipate, ranging from the cost of prescriptions, special diets, and child care to frequent commutes to the hospital for treatments—all on top of your normal everyday living costs. Your financial difficulties won't be solved easily, but hav-

THE QUESTION DOCTOR SAYS:

These Best Questions were written with you, the breast cancer patient, in mind, but they work equally well for couples with joint households. If you feel you can't cope with these financial questions because of everything else going on, ask for help from your partner or find a Certified Financial Planner.

ing a heart-to-heart talk with yourself is a great first step in your money checkup. Cicily Carson Maton, a Certified Financial Planner in Chicago, says, "Emotional distress and lack of financial knowledge will impair your ability to make decisions."

These next 10 Best Questions will help you navigate the rapids. You might also use these questions as the starting point for having talks with your partner or family about money concerns. These Best Questions will keep you focused and take some of the scare out of financial unknowns, as well as give you "permission" to discuss thorny money issues with yourself, your partner, or your family.

⟩⟩⟩THE 10 BEST QUESTIONS
for Financial Health After Breast Cancer

1. What are my financial assets (paper worth and tangible properties)?

The term "financial asset" means anything you own that has monetary value. Financial assets generally refer to what you own on paper, like accounts and funds. Other assets include tangible property such as your house (if you own it) and the vehicles sitting in your driveway.

When you are writing down all your assets, make sure you don't forget to list these major assets:

- Home and real ...
- Other savings
- Insurance policies
- Cash
- Cars, trucks, boats, and motorcycles
- Other valuables, such as appraised collectibles, antiques, and personal property

2. How much money do I have in liquid assets, and where can I get more if I need it?

A liquid asset is any item of value that can be quickly and easily turned into cash. Knowing that you have a potential safety net will help calm your financial fears. Write down your liquid assets or note them separately on your asset list from Best Question 1 above.

The best examples of liquid assets besides cash are certificate of deposits (CDs) and money market accounts. You can cash these in with minimal or no financial penalties. All publicly traded stocks, mutual funds, the cash value in insurance policies, IRAs, and college savings accounts can be liquidated on short notice if need be. There may be some severe tax and social/family penalties in liquidating some of these assets, but if the need arises, they are available. Financial experts suggest you discuss prioritizing your assets so you'll know which to access first, taking tax liabilities and other issues into account.

Antique furniture, real estate, boats, and star-studded baseball card collections are not liquid assets in the truest definition of the term because they take time to sell. Collectibles or other items that you can sell on eBay or at a local yard sale can provide you with cash later on if you need it. You may not be happy about the prospect of selling your grandmother's china, your antique cupboard, or an old doll collection, but at least be aware of your options.

3. What are my debts and expenses?

Creating and living within a budget is a necessary evil—even for financial wizards and Wall Street superstars. You are in good company.

Certified Financial Planner Norman Berk comments, "A budget can help keep you out of debt as well as provide for a means to reduce existing debt. It also can be the focal point for serious review of expenditures so a plan can be developed to have the extra funds if they are suddenly necessary." The first step to managing your personal finances is to identify how you've spent your money in the past. Your debts may already be under control, but chances are they aren't—or at least they're less than ideal. Regardless of your current debt status, be aware that unexpected medical bills are one of the most common reasons people declare personal bankruptcies.

When you are writing down all your debts, make sure you don't forget to list these major expenses:

- Mortgage payment or rent
- Credit card payments
- Auto loans
- Personal loans
- Child care expenses or child-support payments
- Insurance costs
- Living expenses including food, clothing, utilities, fuel,

transportation, parking, cable and Internet charges, personal care, routine medical care (doctor, dentists, and drugs), home repair, entertainment, hobbies, school tuition, magazine/newspaper subscriptions, taxes, vacations, holidays, and other miscellaneous costs

Look into software tools to help you calculate your expenses and plan a budget. There's a free calculator at cgi.money.cnn.com/tools/budget101/budget_101.jsp, as well as commercial personal-finance programs such as Microsoft Money and Quicken.

Get your FICO score if you don't already know it. A FICO score is based on your credit history and is widely used to determine if you are a good credit risk. FICO scores (an acronym for the Fair Isaac Corporation, a Minnesota company that provides numbers to consumers for a fee at www.myfico.com) range from a low of 300 to a perfect 850. Don't go nuts over this exercise, but don't skip it either. The more you understand your current financial status, the better prepared you'll be for any onslaught of new medical bills resulting from your breast cancer care.

If you get into serious debt because of your reduced income and higher expenses, seek help as soon as possible. Don't panic or ignore the situation. Let your creditors know about your cancer.

4. What is my health insurance coverage for my treatments and other medical bills related to my diagnosis?

Breast cancer imposes a heavy financial burden on both patients and their families. For many people, a portion of their medical expenses is paid by their health insurance plan. For individuals who don't have health insurance or who need financial assistance to cover health-care costs, resources are available, including government-sponsored programs and services supported by voluntary organizations.

If you have a health-insurance policy or are covered through your employer, get a copy of your policy as soon as possible and read it carefully to familiarize yourself with the details of your coverage. Take insurance cards with you to all appointments. Everyone involved in the medical care of your breast cancer (health-care providers, hospitals, pharmacies, and laboratories) will need them.

To sidestep costly surprises, talk to your doctor or facility about whether they accept your particular insurance. Then talk to your insurance carrier before you start your treatments about what coverage is available under your policy. Try to get a clear idea of what your out-of-pocket costs will be, although it may be difficult to know the exact amount at this point.

Start asking specific questions about the details of your coverage. For example, find out what your insurance co-pay and deductibles are for in-network and out-of-network providers, how much it will cost you if your doctor doesn't take your insurance, if there is a payment cap, any special rules for cancer, and what kind of preapproval or notification your insurance carrier requires to make sure services are covered.

Financial planner Norman Berk is active with breast cancer community service, and both he and his wife are cancer survivors. He says, "One of your early questions should be about the portability of your insurance

squeaky wheel gets the grease. If you are denied coverage, many financial experts advise that you should complain and agitate for an appeal.

Insurance problems are widespread. If you have health insurance, you might think you'll be covered. But today, many cancer patients with health insurance and even with cancer policies lack sufficient coverage to pay for their treatments. The last place you want to end up is in insurance limbo land or the poorhouse.

5. Do I want to take leave from work, or would I be happier if I continued working? What leave, medical benefits, and schedule flexibility can I reasonably expect from my employer? How many days can I afford to be out?

You must decide soon about taking time off from work during your breast cancer treatments. Your diagnosis, treatment plan, and doctors' advice will largely determine how much time away from work you'll need (if any).

Beyond your doctors' recommendations, you are likely to have some options about how you want to spend your time. Some women choose to devote all their energies to healing. Going back to work may be a difficult step when you contemplate your normal work-related stresses on top of treatment-related side effects and dealing with nosy coworkers. Others prefer to work as a good distraction. Your job may give you something to think about besides your health, make you feel like you have more control over your life, and reconnect you with people who care about you. How the treatments are affecting you will also impact your decision.

For some, the need to keep their incomes drives all else. You may be compelled to work in order not to lose revenue. Another consideration is your partner's or loved one's lost income while he or she is caring for you and taking you to treatment appointments.

If you decide to take time off during the course of your treatment, remember that the U.S. Family and Medical Leave Act allows most workers twelve weeks of leave each year for a serious illness such as breast cancer. You don't necessarily have to take all your leave at once, and you may prefer to dole it out to coincide with your scheduled treatments and posttreatment recovery times.

You can't be discriminated against because of your illness. Most employees are protected by the Americans with Disabilities Act (ADA). Cancer is considered a disability for the purposes of this law. This means that your employer can't treat you any differently from other employees of your company and must make reasonable accommodations if needed. It's comforting to know that legally you can't lose your job because of your absence or illness.

6. How well organized are my personal financial papers, accounts, and records?

Managing financial records, medical bills, and routine bills is a challenge for most people. A lot of people resist creating filing systems because it's too boring. Other people relish taming their paper-clutter monsters.

Whatever your organizational style, you are about to meet new challenges. You can prevent unnecessary stress and financial crises by keeping accurate and well-organized files related to your insurance claims and benefits, including letters of medical necessity, bills, receipts, requests for sick leave, and correspondence with insurance companies.

One simple subquestion ... ...

...suggests setting up automated online accounts. A financial planner, attorney, bookkeeper, or CPA can also help you to get your personal finances organized and suggest ways to stay organized, too.

7. Have I designated a financial power of attorney? Do I have a medical power of attorney? Do I have a legally binding document stating who this person or persons are?

Taking care of this business is hard. But as painful as it might be to think like this and take these recommended actions, consider this legal protection as an act of generosity and kindness—as well as necessity. You are lifting the burden of difficult decisions from those you love. According to Cicily Carson Maton, "A power of attorney for health is very important to have in place so your agent can pay your bills and take care of your affairs. It is absolutely vital."

Many perfectly healthy partners have active financial powers of attorney for each other in case something happens to one of them. This document gives your partner or another trusted person broad authority to handle your finances if you can't. A "durable" power of attorney won't automatically end if you become incapacitated. A lawyer can assist you, or check the Nolo Web site (www.nolo.com) for more details.

A medical power of attorney is a separate but similar document that specifies your wishes if you become medically incapacitated. Consider getting this document prepared before any surgeries or long-distance travel for treatments. Your hospital or clinic may provide this form for free, but it's best to check with a lawyer or financial planner for his final blessing.

8. Do I have an estate plan and a will? Are my other legal affairs in order?

Estate planning is the orderly process of preparing to transfer your affairs and assets to your intended beneficiaries. A good estate plan should also minimize taxes, court costs, and attorney's fees, while addressing your own welfare and needs. Most adults need an estate plan regardless of the size of their estates. You should, at the very least, legally designate your partner or another trusted loved one as the person who will manage your financial affairs.

A will is not just for rich people. No matter how much or how little money you have, a will helps to ensure that your children and other beneficiaries will not suffer undue confusion or anxiety about your wishes for them. If you don't have a will, state law will determine who gets your property, and a judge may decide who will raise your children. Making a will doesn't require much legal knowledge, but you have a lot of personal decisions to make. Depending on the size and complexity of your estate (second marriages, children, stepchildren, etc.), you may need legal assistance for creating or updating your will. Another alternative is legal software such as Quicken WillMaker Plus to help you create a living will, a living trust, a financial power of attorney, and other legal documents. A living will (also called a living trust or medical directive) gives you the opportunity to declare your intentions about lifesaving efforts on your behalf and to appoint a representative to ensure your intentions are followed.

get int. If you have a financial advisor or plan to hire one, she can help you with planning these documents.

For example, an unanticipated financial worry for breast cancer patients is the burden of extra costs at Christmas/holiday time. A study found that 66 percent of cancer patients worry how they will afford Christmas on top of their medical bills. More than half the people in this study said they were cutting back on Christmas presents as a way to ease spending concerns.

> *If you didn't have a financial advisor prior to your diagnosis, reach out to those people around you whom you trust and ask for their help in sorting through the financial issues.*
>
> —CICILY CARSON MATON, CERTIFIED FINANCIAL PLANNER

So the short version of the short answer is to find ways to cut back on your expenses and understand your own "financial footprint." Clarify what is important to you. Start by looking at your spending habits as honestly as possible. Here are some red flags from the National Foundation for Credit Counseling for poor money management:

- Always late with bill payments
- Withdrawn funds from your retirement or savings accounts to pay current expenses
- Calls from creditors about overdue bills
- Credit card cash advances to pay off other creditors

- Minimum repayments on installment charges
- Overtime work to make ends meet

10. Who can I turn to for financial help in a worst-case scenario (no insurance, lose my job, spent my life savings, etc.)?

During your cancer treatments you are working with a medical team of doctors, nurses, and technicians, each with his own role in your care. Similarly, you need to assemble a financial team of family members, experts and advisors (including a lawyer, financial planner, CPA, and estate planner), supporters, and cheerleaders.

The ideal quarterback of this financial team is a Certified Financial Planner. A financial planner looks at the big picture of your money matters as well as advises you on bills, income, insurance, taxes, and investments. A skillful planner can help you develop a plan to repay medical bills and rebuild your bank account. He might have solutions you never thought of. Financial planner Norman Berk comments, "It's hard to find the time to make a sound financial plan, and the task of finding a reputable planner might seem too daunting right now. Yet planning has its rewards." Consider asking your caregiver or partner to take on the role of finding a financial planner you can work with. Some specialize in helping people with chronic illnesses. Ideally, make this contact as soon as possible.

Aside from getting professional help, think about people you know from whom you could borrow money if needed and what other assets might serve as collateral for a loan. By thinking about the worst-case scenario, you may actually feel more prepared to face whatever comes.

You and your family can discuss financial concerns with a medical social worker or the business office at your hospital or clinic. A hospital social worker is often a good source for advice and referrals on handling your medical bills.

...assistance for cancer patients. Check with the American Cancer Society (www.cancer.org) and the National Cancer Institute (www.cancer.gov) for complete lists of organizations and for available options for uninsured breast cancer patients.

- **CancerCare,** a national nonprofit agency, offers free financial assistance; www.cancercare.org.
- **Cancer Legal Resource Center** provides free phone advice on insurance and cancer-related legal issues; www.lls.edu/academics/candp/clrc.html.
- **Cancer Supportive Care** has information on pharmaceutical reimbursement assistance programs available through drug manufacturers; www.cancersupportivecare.com/drug_assistance.html.
- **National Foundation for Credit Counseling** is a nonprofit that offers free and low-cost debt counseling, education, and planning advice (see its online tool Instant Budget Maker); http://cgi.money.cnn.com/tools/instant-budget/instantbudget_101.jsp.
- **National Patient Travel Center** for financially-strapped patients who need to travel long distances for treatment; www.patienttravel.org/.
- **Patient Advocate Foundation** offers free counseling on managed care, insurance, financial issues, job discrimination, and debt; www.patientadvocate.org.

There might be financial relief on the horizon you don't know about.

❯ Ask if your doctor or hospital offers interest-free installment payment plans.

❯ Check the fine print on your auto loan, mortgage, and credit cards for disability insurance coverage which most people aren't aware of.

❯ Negotiate doctor bills, hospital bills, and insurance claims (or ask a loved one or financial professional to negotiate on your behalf).

❯ Investigate health-insurance risk pools, special programs created by state legislatures as a safety net for the "medically uninsurable" population.

❯ Consider a fundraising event within your family, community, or religious group to help you pay bills.

❯ The Magic Question

What would I really like to splurge on?

Time to channel your inner shopper. You need to treat yourself well and counteract all those worries about your diagnosis and money. Maybe a little trip down the shoe aisle, finding a dazzling new handbag, lighting a new set of scented candles, or snuggling with your partner at a romantic bed and breakfast might be just what the doctor should have ordered.

If you can afford a little spending spree without breaking the bank, go for it. Think of your purchase as "comfort food." You'll feel more human again and stronger for your upcoming war on breast cancer.

CONCLUSION

Women are historically worse off financially than men, with many giving up work to raise children, thus having a smaller pension and savings. They are also less li~~kel~~ ~~~~ ~~~~

~~~~ with them more proactively if you take the time now to assess your situation and figure out how to locate financial assistance if needed. When that's done you can really focus your energies on getting well, and you won't be trying to fight financial fatigue and insurance exhaustion at the same time.

THE 10 BEST RESOURCES

American Cancer Society. "Medical Insurance and Financial Assistance for the Cancer Patient." www.cancer.org/docroot/MLT/content/MLT_1x_Medical_Insurance_and_Financial_Assistance_for_the_Cancer_Patient.asp?sitearea=&level=1.

Angel Foundation. "Financial Assistance." foundation.mohpa.com/cancer_financial_assistance.html.

CancerCare. "Financial Help for People with Cancer." www.cancercare.org/pdf/fact_sheets/fs_financial_en.pdf.

Healthwell Foundation. "Helping Patients Afford Medical Treatments." www.healthwellfoundation.org/index.aspx.

HOPE Guide. "Cancer-Related Financial Assistance and Access to Cancer Screenings." www.hopeguide.org.

Landay, David S. *Be Prepared: The Complete Financial, Legal and Practical Guide for Living with a Life-Challenging Condition.* New York: St. Martin's Press, 1998.

National Cancer Institute. "Fact Sheet: Financial Assistance and Other Resources for People With Cancer." www.cancer.gov/cancertopics/factsheet/Support/financial-resources.

Patient Access Network Foundation. "How to Apply" (for financial assistance). www.patientaccessnetwork.org/HowApply.aspx.

Patient Advocate Foundation. "Resources for Solving Insurance and Healthcare Problems." www.patientadvocate.org.

Willis, Clint. "On the Road to Financial Health." *Money Magazine*, October 1, 2006. money.cnn.com/magazines/moneymag/moneymag_archive/2006/10/01/8387559/index.htm.

poet

Breast cancer will almost surely have a profound effect on your marriage or long-term partnership. A diagnosis of breast cancer can magnify a relationship's past imperfections and strengthen what was already strong between partners.

Rarely does breast cancer cause a divorce or separation. Stories perpetually circulate about the baddest of bad husbands—those bums who walk out on their wife of twenty years, leaving her to deal with the kids, chemotherapy, and a mountain of medical bills. But the statistics say fortunately that this "Hall of Shameful Husbands," so named by Marc Silver in his book, *Breast Cancer Husband,* is actually quite small.

Typically, relationships that were strong before the diagnosis of breast cancer remain strong after surgery and treatment. Jennie Nash, author of *The Victoria's Secret Catalog Never Stops Coming, and Other Lessons I Learned from Breast Cancer*, recalls her own situation: "A breast cancer diagnosis magnifies everything in your life. So if your marriage's not good, then it's going to magnify that. I was lucky because what was magnified was really great . . . he behaved as if it was his cancer, too." Dave Balch, husband of breast cancer survivor Chris, speaks from his personal experience: "What cancer does is it tends to make strong marriages stronger and weak marriages weaker. If there's a problem in the marriage that gets intensified, it's probably because the marriage isn't as strong as you think.

In a strong marriage, all that other stuff is just crap and it goes away." Win Boerckel, an oncology social worker for the cancer support organization CancerCare, has counseled hundreds of couples. He comments, "Usually cancer doesn't create better bonding and communications in troubled marriages."

Communication breakdowns happen because there is often a dramatic shift of roles in the partnership. Daily routines are heaved upside down, almost like an earthquake has rocked your home. Both partners feel tremendous stress, usually within their relationship as well as from external stressors like treatments, schedules, and financial worries.

Many studies of relationships touched by cancer universally confirm that in general men and women truly communicate about and deal with cancer differently. The male brain is hardwired to solve problems and be a Mr. Fix-it. So it drives guys crazy when they can't "fix" their partner's breast cancer. This results in a tremendous sense of powerlessness, frustration, and failure for men, which often goes underappreciated by the woman, who is on overload already in her battle against breast cancer.

But the real challenge for men is to learn how to be the caregiver that his partner needs, not what he thinks she needs—a problem solver. Some men grease their relationships for years with offers of sex, dinner dates, occasional romantic getaways, and roses on Valentine's Day. This works fine until breast cancer hits. The male partner must suddenly learn all about a terribly complicated disease, go on lots of appointments and juggle work-home priorities while still having his own life to manage. Most men care deeply about their loved ones with breast cancer. But often these new demands hit them hard at the very same moment they find themselves thrust into the often unfamiliar role of being a primary caregiver.

The other key difference between men and women is their comfort with the role of caregiver. Women are traditionally the nurtur-

THE QUESTION

...ₑₑ ₛ ₘₒᵣₑ good advice from Harriette Cole, author of the nationally syndicated advice column "Sense and Sensitivity" and the creative director of *Ebony* magazine. "It's best in the beginning to ask welcoming questions. Do your best not to be hostile or condescending or doubting or in any way negative in your questions . . . Ask your questions honestly and without judgment and not like an inquisition."

ers in their households. After breast cancer, many men find they must become caregivers, yet they don't know how. This lack of practice combined with a sense of urgency and inadequacy can lead to great frustrations and misunderstandings.

The goal of this chapter is to help you and your partner communicate better by asking each other the following Best Questions. These questions will work in either direction—the patient asking her partner or the partner asking the patient—and will work for all couples, including patients in lesbian relationships. Revisit these Best Questions over time in addition to discussing them after the initial diagnosis to help you to understand how your relationship is changing and where your current needs are.

IF YOU LOVE SOMEONE WITH BREAST CANCER

If the woman you love has been diagnosed with breast cancer, it's important that you remain at her side and become an integral part of her healing. You may be experiencing many conflicting emotions right now. That's OK and that's normal.

Your understandable desires to be knowledgeable and protective may be causing you guilt and frustrations that you aren't fully acknowledging. You may also be feeling anger, denial, a sense of betrayal, and even thinking about your own mortality. Most of the Best Questions in chapter 14 on coping with emotions will work for you, too, so try them for yourself.

Just as women with breast cancer go through emotional upheavals and cycles, studies conducted with breast cancer husbands and partners found that they have a variety of problems, including eating and sleeping disorders. One of the most positive ways to channel your energies and need to help is to do research on breast cancer for your partner. Becoming informed is a powerful tool in fighting a sense of helplessness and confusion. You can be the one to search the Internet, read books, and find resources for support. Just be savvy about how much new information your partner can deal with at any given time, since she's probably feeling overwhelmed and tired, too.

>>> THE 10 BEST QUESTIONS
When Talking with Your Partner

1. When were we most successful in communicating with each other in the past? How can we use the same methods now to deal with this illness together?

Breast cancer is the newest member of your family, a most unwanted and uninvited houseguest who's here to stay. Your communication becomes more critical than ever. One way to start this conversation and not feel overwhelmed by the current circumstances is to reflect on past times that you two communicated well. Talk over these times, remember how ...

... you are navigating uncharted waters such as breast cancer. It's better to talk in specifics, keep open a free exchange of ideas, and not only express your feelings, but also "own" them. One way to do this is to use frequent "I" and "we" messages ("I

point. That's never the end of the point, she's just warming up.

—DR. JOHN GRAY, RELATIONSHIP GURU AND AUTHOR OF THE BEST-SELLING BOOK SERIES, *MEN ARE FROM MARS, WOMEN ARE FROM VENUS*

think we should . . ." "I feel we need to consider . . .").

Another way both partners can be better listeners is to use paraphrasing, or reflecting back what the other said to clarify the meaning and show you were attentive. Relationship experts recommend using openers like, "I hear you saying . . . Is that right?" or "Tell me more." Your body language—making eye contact, sitting close by, and keeping your facial expressions open and positive—also goes a long way in smoothing your communications. Be sure to ask each other questions as they come up.

2. What areas of our lives must we maintain to ensure as much normalcy as possible?

When breast cancer moves into your home—regardless of what life was like for you prior to your diagnosis and where you are now on your cancer journey—you must still keep some semblance of normalcy in order to function on a daily basis.

Solve this problem together as a team. Your life and household

FOR LESBIAN WOMEN WHO LOVE SOMEONE WITH BREAST CANCER

Coming Out About Lesbians and Cancer, a research report conducted by the Lesbians and Breast Cancer Project Team for the Ontario Breast Cancer Community Research Initiative in 2004, concluded with some key findings for lesbians who have been touched by cancer.

Lesbian breast cancer patients reported feeling strongly supported by their partners. But in a lesbian relationship there is at least one additional twist—the partner is likely to think, "It could be me." This worked both for and against lesbians. It made partners more empathetic, since they know their own breasts, too. Other times, the partner physically and emotionally identified with the patient in ways that made support awkward or extremely difficult. Lorraine Biros, director of client services at the Mautner Project: The National Lesbian Health Organization in Washington, D.C., says, "There's a fear factor for lesbians. The well partner sometimes asks herself, 'Will I be next?' "

The fear of cancer causes breakdowns in dialogue both within relationships and within the lesbian community. Lesbians with breast cancer may feel especially isolated because they often lack the institutional support that heterosexual couples take for granted—the social support of accepting family members and legal and financial recognition. For lesbians, being public about their cancer often parallels the experience of coming out as a lesbian.

As happens in heterosexual partnerships, lesbians' worries include concerns about sexual performance and still being seen as desirable. The Best Questions in this chapter are generic enough to be useful for lesbians finding their way along their cancer journeys.

Resources and support for lesbian couples include:

> Lesbian Community Cancer Project; www.lccp.org

> Lesbians with Cancer, About.com; www.lesbianlife.about.com

> The Mautner Project: The National Lesbian Health Organization; www.mautnerproject.org

> Lesbian Cancer Initiative; www.gaycenter.org/program_folders/LCI/program_view

> Lesbian.com; www.lesbian.com/health/health_intro.html

responsibilities must ...

... long-distance friends, for example, might belong into your "Have to Have" bucket rather than your "Nice to Have" bucket.

3. What role changes in our partnership do we need to make to get through this thing together?

Your past roles and the division of labor in your partnership may be turned upside down after a diagnosis of breast cancer. In essence, you have two new job descriptions to write. This is a critical task that should not be overlooked or shoved under the rug. The reason is that couples' misunderstandings and unspoken assumptions about roles are a breeding ground for festering guilt, resentments, and potentially lifelong animosities toward each other.

You and your partner need an early discussion on roles to clarify expectations as soon on the cancer journey as possible. The man might have to cook or at least pick up the carryout dinners. He might be assuming that his wife wants him to do everything around the house or all the routine chores. However, this is typically where lots of independent women get feisty.

From the patient's perspective, she feels her sense of control and personal freedom is jeopardized by the very acts of kindness her partner thinks he's performing on her behalf. "Women are not used to having people take care of them," says oncology social worker Pat Spicer. "They can't decide how to handle it."

Dave Balch recalls the moment the light bulb went on in his male mind while talking with his wife, Chris:

> We chose to have our treatment one hundred miles from here and I did all the driving. And Chris said to me, "You know, it's really bugging me that you're doing all the driving right now." Whoa! I thought I was being helpful . . . She told me that she felt like she had no control over anything. So I said, "What do you want to do," and she said, "Let me drive to the bottom of the mountain and then you can drive." This is an example of the importance of being able to communicate. She needed to be able to tell me that without me exploding on her.

Whenever one partner gets sick, a couple's usual pattern of give-and-take, dependence and independence, is altered. Breast cancer can bring a couple closer together; it can also uncover shortcomings in the relationship.

4. What has this been like for you?

This simple question, suggested by Pat Spicer, may uncover a hornet's nest of complaints, a flood of feelings, or no new information at all. She says, "Women are often caught up in their own feelings and never hear what the other person is going through." In fact, often it's the couples that assume they already know each other well that get the biggest surprises. Relationship advisors Dr. Scott Peck and Shannon Peck of Solana Beach, California, commented, "There are many ways to bring the empowering combination of kindness and love into your marriage. One way is to ask simple direct questions . . . this can bring great healing power."

Breast cancer survivor Betty Rollin commented recently on the value of simple questions. "The best question a partner or friend or anyone can ask a patient is simply, 'How are you'—and sound as if you mean it . . . Then the patient can open up or not, but the important thing is that interest and caring have been shown." This

control. In Dave Balch's story above, he thought that his driving was easing the stress on his wife Chris, but being treated with kid gloves was actually stressing her out even more.

Many couples experience internal misunderstandings, self-pity, misdirected anger, and financial and sexual problems after a diagnosis of breast cancer. The only way out is to work together as a team. Identify what's causing each of you the greatest stress and then talk over what you can do to alleviate some of the stress. For the patient, this is a great time to learn how to ask for help. For the partner, this is a great time to organize a "help posse": create a list of tasks that need doing, like picking up dry cleaning, shopping, running errands, or paying bills, and match the tasks with a list of people who have volunteered their time and services.

The partner can activate his "help posse" when someone calls or e-mails and sincerely wants to help out. He'll be ready with an answer like, "Well, sure, we actually could really use someone to mail a package for us tomorrow." There are also commercial and free Web sites and sources to help you organize these arrangements. Ask your local social worker or your support group for more suggestions.

6. How can I show you that I love you?

Marc Silver describes the male perspective in his book *Breast Cancer Husband.* "Start by telling your wife that you love her. These are words that are sometimes hard to say, sometimes easy to say. But no one can say them in the same way that you can. And there's never been a better time to say them."

Regardless how sexy each of you is feeling these days, there's always time and reason to give each other hugs. Be a "love pharmacist" and dispense your hugs like good medicine.

If hugging just isn't your thing, then what is? Besides saying, "I love you," find a way to show your love for each other on a daily basis. A card of encouragement, a phone call, a back rub, or a special meal are all small things that mean so much when you are not up to par or are an overworked caregiver.

7. How can we still enjoy being together and have fun?

Your breast cancer hasn't robbed you of your sense of humor or your need to have a bit of fun once in a while. Sure, you probably can't do all the things you could before, but that doesn't mean you can't do anything that's fun or at least talk about doing it after your treatments are over.

What's something silly or easy that you two can do together once in a while just like the old days before breast cancer moved in at your place? Go get your favorite take-out Chinese food or pizza, watch a stupid movie together, take a hike together, or see old friends who know you well enough to not bring up your cancer.

You don't want to live in a world devoid of humor and lighthearted news. Just because the patient is sick and cancer is serious, it still doesn't give you both a license to be deadly serious all the time.

Being sick is no fun, and you don't have to pretend it's okay when it's not. At the same time, laughter is the best medicine and can go a long way in strengthening the good glue of your relationship.

know what to do to help.' "

Asking for help is often the breast cancer patient's biggest challenge and hardest lesson to learn. Most women are raised to be caregivers, not care receivers. Now it's time to shift roles and ask for help with anything that can be done by someone else. The basic disconnect is between the woman who doesn't have much practice in asking for help and the man who doesn't have much practice in giving help except to solve problems, which we've already agreed won't work with cancer.

By asking each other this question, you'll have a chance to talk out these differences and explore areas of agreement and mutual needs.

9. Do we need professional counseling or other help for our marriage?

A sign of strength is knowing when you need outside help to overcome your differences or communication breakdowns. There is nothing to be ashamed of if you decide you need marriage counseling, want to join a support group, or decide to meet with a therapist. Ideally, seek a professional with a specific background in helping couples touched by cancer. Ask a local social worker, your doctor, or a nurse navigator for suggested names.

If you are interested in joining a support group, see chapter 15 for advice and Best Questions. Below is a list of national support groups for partners that may also help you. Also try your hospital or doctor for suggestions of support groups for partners.

- BreastCancer.org; www.breastcancer.org
- The Mautner Project: The National Lesbian Health Organization; www.mautnerproject.org
- OncoChat; www.oncochat.org
- Association of Cancer Online Resources; www.acor.org
- Men Against Breast Cancer; www.menagainstbreastcancer.org
- Well Spouse Association; www.wellspouse.org

10. What old rules do we need to break? What new rules do we need to establish?

Most relationships have unwritten but inviolable rules that govern everything from who takes the garbage out to how nutritious dinner has to be. This is the opposite of Best Question 2 above about normalcy and what *not* to change. Now we're talking about what you *do* want to change in your postdiagnosis world.

Your old rules are probably pretty simple, even if you've never exactly thought of them before as rules. Typically, rules have to do with household chores (who does what and when), favorite routines that may need permission (playing Friday night poker with the boys or shopping sprees with the girls), and the little picky stuff (how neatly the laundry gets folded and where to put the bowls in the dishwasher).

Families with children often also have rules revolving around what the children can and can't do based on requirements like doing their math homework, piano practice, or finishing all their green beans at dinner. Some rules come from how we were raised, and others just evolve over time.

Now it's time to figure out together which rules to let go of and

source of unspoken assumptions and subsequent misunderstandings between partners. One way to avoid arguments is to call a truce on judging each other's past actions and rules. In fact, the very best new rule is to agree to wipe the slate clean and start over again—as a team.

❯ The Magic Question

What are you afraid to ask me? What are we not talking about that needs to be addressed?

This is the all-important "elephant in the room" question. Having an elephant in the room means that everyone present is ignoring an obvious truth and not talking about something right under their noses.

So, what is *your* elephant? Most likely, your elephant is something you're intensely afraid of, like facing your own mortality, your repulsion to seeing a disfigured breast, lost sexual intimacy, or unspoken worries about family finances.

Unacknowledged elephants have a way of just getting bigger and bigger unless you point them out and admit to their existence. This might be a hard question to ask each other. But with the right spirit of shared hopes and dreams, it can be the most liberating question you ever ask.

THE 10 BEST QUESTIONS FOR SEXUAL HEALTH AND INTIMACY AFTER BREAST CANCER

Sex may have been the last thing on your mind after your diagnosis of breast cancer. Most women become very focused on survival, their treatment options, and all the anxieties that go into learning about breast cancer as they deal with their many decisions and uncertainties. But being intimate can make you feel loved and supported as you go through your cancer treatments and live your life beyond being a breast cancer patient. Resuming sexual relations and intimacy might even help you move from being a breast cancer patient to becoming a breast cancer survivor.

Some sex experts say that your most potent—and most underutilized—sex tool is your voice. Asking each other these Best Questions, along with your own personal questions, will get you started on rekindling sexual desire. You'll learn how your partner feels, what he or she wants, and how to make each other happy.

1. **How can we best communicate with each other about our needs for sex and intimacy?**
   Women tend to romanticize sex and intimacy, while men are more likely to have a body-centered or recreational approach to sexual encounters. These natural differences between men and women explain why talking about sex and intimacy can be tricky. In their book *Intimacy after Cancer: A Woman's Guide,* Sally Kydd and Dana Rowett comment, "Men don't ask for directions and don't read instructions . . . even for sex. Just show us the parts, and we'll put it together."

   Your best communications on sex might be using no words at all. Perhaps having some signals or a couple of phrases can serve as "code" for when one of you is feeling amorous. Working out your personal preferences and communication styles in advance can help smooth out misunderstandings and clarify expectations.

2. **Are you comfortable being intimate again?**
   It's possible that nothing can prepare either of you for the shock of what your chest looks like after surgery. Examine and touch the scars together to help you both adjust to the physical changes. Scars will heal over time and become less red and raw looking. If you engage in sex, the partner may fear hurting the patient during lovemaking. Talk with the patient about the sexual positions that are the most comfortable for her. The partner should also

Even though the partner understands this at one level, it's also quite common for the partner to still feel rejected, resentful, and drained from his or her caregiving demands. Here are some suggestions for things to try from experts in cancer and sexuality:

> Enjoy a romantic candlelit dinner.

> Offer a long sensual massage.

> Watch an erotic video together.

> Try new sexual positions.

> Book a romantic vacation or quick get-away trip.

4. **For the partner to ask: What do you want to tell me about the physical changes in your body?**
   This is a very direct question about a topic many couples avoid discussing. Women may hesitate to share their pain or feelings about their new appearance, fearing they will alienate their partners. Male partners may be reluctant to discuss the woman's physical changes because it's a constant reminder of how powerless they have been to "fix the cancer," a nearly universal male reaction.

5. **What can I do to please you?**
   Become dedicated to recapturing mutual pleasure for you and your partner. Sex is fun and pleasure is good medicine for the patient — and for your relationship.

6. **What's the craziest or funniest thing we could do to show our love for each other?**
   Rediscover your passion by having fun together. Go from boring or scared to blissful in the bedroom. Be creative with your passion and direct it toward your partner with a renewed fire. Nurture it. Enjoy and revel in it. You are alive.

(continued)

7. **Is there anything off-limits now that was okay before?**

   If you don't ask each other this question, your unspoken assumptions about what's acceptable and what isn't can lead to major misunderstandings. Be clear about your limits and nonjudgmental about your partner's desires. Talk this question out without criticism or bringing up your past sexual or marital problems.

8. **We agree we both have a low interest in sex right now. What can we do to get back on track?**

   This Best Question is for circumstances when you both have a low sex drive and agree that this is a shared situation. You may end up agreeing that neither of you wants to resume sexual relations for a while. This might be your new definition of "back on track," but at least you've made sure you both agree with it.

9. **We can't agree about having sexual relations or being intimate. How can we work it out?**

   Keep in mind that even if your sexual desire is reduced or absent it's still possible to be a good lover. During this time, you still can be physically intimate without sexual intercourse through kissing, touching, stroking, cuddling, hugging, massaging, or sharing loving words.

10. **Do we need professional help?**

    Sexual problems create emotional problems and vice versa. You may want to talk to a professional therapist or counselor, ideally as a couple. There are many professionally trained specialists who deal with intimacy and sexuality issues for cancer patients and their partners. Ask an oncology social worker or a nurse navigator for a referral. Some large cancer care centers have specialists connected to their facility.

The Magic Question

What are you afraid to ask me about in our sexual relationship? What sexual fears are we not talking about that need to be addressed?

Not talking about sexual problems or your fears puts a tremendous strain on your relationship, just at the very time when you need closeness, good communications, and each other's support to get through the cancer journey together.

and your relationship will grow and strengthen. Ideally, couples should go through the entire process—diagnosis, treatment, and recovery—as loving partners in an open dialogue, not two people pulled apart by fear of the unknown. Maintaining strong communications is essential. Silence may be misinterpreted as a lack of interest or caring.

Asking each other these 10 Best Questions and any of your own "best questions" as they occur to you will enrich your communications, clear the air, and help you and your partner enjoy a healthy and happy relationship together. Fears, stress, and anger are best extinguished by honest sharing and "best listening," too.

THE 10 BEST RESOURCES

American Cancer Society. "Caring for the Patient with Cancer at Home: A Guide for Patients and Families." www.cancer.org/docroot/MBC/MBC_2x_OtherEffects.asp.

American Cancer Society. "Sexuality for Women and Their Partners." www.cancer.org/docroot/MIT/MIT_7_1x_SexualityforWomenandTheir Partners.asp.

Carr, Kris. "Bandage or Bondage: Dating, Sex, Marriage, Babies," in *Crazy Sexy Cancer Tips*. Guilford, CT: Globe Pequot Press, 2007.

Gray, John. *Men Are from Mars, Women Are from Venus: The Classic Guide to Understanding the Opposite Sex*. New York: Harper Paperbacks, 2004.

Mautner Project, the National Lesbian Health Organization. "Programs and Services." www.mautnerproject.org.

Men Against Breast Cancer. "For the Women We Love: A Breast Cancer Battle Plan." www.menagainstbreastcancer.org.

National Cancer Institute. "Dealing with a New Self-Image." www.cancer.gov/cancertopics/takingtime/page7.

National Cancer Institute. "Taking Time: Support for People with Cancer." www.cancer.gov/cancertopics/takingtime/page6#E4.

National Cancer Institute. "When Someone You Love Is Being Treated for Cancer." www.cancer.gov/cancertopics/When-Someone-You-Love-Is-Treated.

Silver, Marc. *Breast Cancer Husband: How to Help Your Wife (and Yourself) Through Diagnosis, Treatment, and Beyond.* Emmaus, PA: Rodale, 2004.

U.S. humorist

Just one generation ago a diagnosis of breast cancer was often a secret shared only among the smallest circle of family members and closest of friends. According to one study, as recently as 1961 only 10 percent of doctors even told their patients that they had breast cancer! Nowadays, the news of yet another friend, co-worker, or aunt with breast cancer is often greeted with the assumption that the more we all talk about it, the better.

But is that really true? Sharing a breast cancer diagnosis with the world isn't as easy—or hard—as it may seem at first. The fact that this is about your breast, an intimate part of your body, also complicates things. As Marion Long, writing in the breast cancer magazine *MAMM,* says, "Some of the women say they now regret all the secrecy, but others feel that their insistence on privacy served them well, and they would choose the same course again."

You may be a naturally extroverted person, someone who announces a diagnosis of breast cancer to the whole world without giving it a second thought either by posting it on your Facebook page, setting up a blog or video cam, broadcasting e-mails to every person in your address book, or by calling your entire Rolodex. On the other hand, perhaps you are a naturally shy and reserved person who prefers to share things with only a very small inner circle—and wouldn't dream of doing it any other way.

If you are one extreme or the other—either very open or very

> *Ladies, this advice may sound fluffy, but it's so helpful . . . before you tell the important people in your life, look your best. Get an eyebrow wax, a manicure, and a new outfit. I call it "Cancer Armor."*
>
> —QUOTED IN *CRAZY SEXY CANCER TIPS* BY KRIS CARR

reserved—then this chapter isn't for you. This is a nonissue, a no-brainer for you. You already have clear preferences about telling others about your diagnosis and already know how you will handle telling your mother, your gym buddy, and the workplace gossip.

On the other hand, if you are somewhere in the middle of this continuum of extroversion and introversion like most people, the decisions surrounding who to tell about your diagnosis of breast cancer might be some of the toughest and most likely to keep you awake at night.

Breast cancer husband Dave Balch emphasizes how important it is to consider carefully whom you want to tell about your breast cancer diagnosis. He says, "Dealing with telling other people is huge and cannot be understated."

Some women debate obsessively about whom they should tell about their breast cancer. Over and over again, they toss this question around and around, imagining the "telling scene," then the other person's reaction, and then their own responses—a full-blown drama of tears, hugs, blame, and pity.

If you are one of these people, this chapter is for you. Ask yourself the following Best Questions as a way to sort through rationally your own needs and priorities about informing people. These questions will help you to resolve internal conflicts about which bucket—the "Tell" bucket or the "Don't Tell" bucket—that best suits the various people in your life. The Question Doctor hopes this chapter helps you to sort out another set of potentially stressful decisions that you face and probably didn't anticipate—whom to tell, when, and how.

>>> THE 10 BEST QUESTIONS
Before Breaking the News to Others

1. In the past when something bad has happened to me, did I find relief and comfort in talking about it or not?

You want to reduce as much unnecessary stress as possible and encourage your own good mental and physical health. Your answer to this soul-searching question will help you understand your own needs for talking about things as a way to resolve issues and find peace.

Think back to your previous tough situations, like boyfriend or husband breakups, the death of a loved one, the time you almost flunked out of school, or when you lost out on a job promotion. What did you do? Did you talk, talk, talk about it to just about anyone who would listen? Or did you share with only your most trusted confidantes? Maybe you sought friendship and solace through online chats or by texting friends.

Licensed clinical oncology social worker Win Boerckel shares insights from his twelve years of counseling cancer patients: "Sometimes people are very private prior to the cancer diagnosis and they just want to maintain that privacy. Some people are very tight on self-disclosure and are uncomfortable in any situation where they have to reveal things about themselves."

In contrast, author Jennie Nash believes that bad news does less damage when it's shared. "I really dreaded someone not knowing. Like running into them and having to go through the whole thing. I wanted to get everyone's grief over with all at the same time instead of having to relive it day after day. I couldn't say that I was fine."

Whatever your style, just know two things. First, there's no right or wrong answer to this question. Second, go with the communication style that best suits you personally, not what someone else would do.

If you naturally crave sociability, or if privacy is your preference, go with whatever has worked best for you in the past. This isn't an all-or-nothing proposition. Some people are naturally easier to tell than others. Best Questions 5 through 10 will help you to decide which specific people you want to tell.

2. Who can I recruit for my "knowledge and feel good" team?

You've already got a medical team and perhaps a financial team to help you get through this diagnosis. Now it's time to ask yourself, "Who do I know who makes me laugh, has already survived chemotherapy, or works in the medical field?" Look around and extend your reach outward to these people who can help you the most based on their expertise, insights, or ability to make you feel good.

It makes sense to confide in people who can give you something of value or provide comfort in return for your confidence. This is a smart strategy and a good use of your valuable time. Knowledge is power. The people you know with direct experience with breast cancer—even if you aren't close to them—can be an invaluable resource. You might be amazed at how willing near-strangers are to share intimate details of their own experiences. Let the sisterhood of breast cancer work to your benefit. Reach out and soak up others' experiences and lessons learned. Other survivors can be your most valuable resource.

In addition, find at least one good f...

... ...u-last rules about secret keeping. She believes that most advice is often too simplistic, focusing on one-size-fits-all solutions, such as "never tell" or "always be completely honest." Sometimes keeping a secret can be appropriate and helpful, but other times it can be harmful. It's up to you to decide which is right for you as you consider your potential list of people.

Most likely your motivations for telling certain people will be based on three things. First, there's your natural tendency to talk or not (see Best Question 1). Second, there are people you feel obligated to tell, those with a real need to know (see Best Question 4). And third, there are people that you choose to tell, either because of your closeness to them or because they will bring you comfort during your healing process. Having outlets for your thoughts and feelings can lift your spirits and ease the load. Maybe you need both quiet time and talk time.

As you sort through your motivations, in some ways it's almost like planning the guest list for your wedding. You can think of all sorts of people you are fond of and want to include in your big wedding day. But then reality takes over as you ask yourself, "Can I really afford to feed this person?" Just like planning a wedding guest list, some borderline people in your life, from workplace acquaintances to the people who only send you annual Christmas cards, will drop off the list and get moved to the "Don't Tell" bucket without consequences either to you or them.

4. Who has a genuine need to know about my diagnosis? Whom am I obligated to tell and when should I tell them?

There'll be obvious people to tell, such as your partner, immediate family members, and close friends. If your children are old enough, you'll feel obligated to tell them. See chapter 19 for the Best Questions for children.

As advanced oncology nurse Melissa Craft says, "The people who love you are going to know. If you make decisions about not including the closest people around you in your diagnosis, you have taken away their right to respond and care for you. This is very controlling."

Most likely you'll need to tell your employer, especially if you ask for extended sick leave from work during your treatments. Best Question 9 in this chapter addresses the issue of telling your employer.

And there are obvious people not to tell, like the convenience store clerk, the stranger sitting next to you on the flight to Denver, and a nosy neighbor or coworker. But most everyone else falls in between. The idea here is to make a list of the people in your life who meet the minimum requirements for the "Tell" bucket. Then decide how, when, and where you'll break the news. It could be that keeping this secret bottled up inside you will take more energy than you realize. It might even cause you to deny your diagnosis and need for immediate surgery and treatments.

5. How will this person most likely react to my diagnosis?

Reactions among your dearest friends and family members are likely to run the gamut from shock to quiet acceptance. But just because someone is close to you doesn't mean they'll react well. Even just the word "cancer" is a fearful word, and some of your closest loved ones may be devastated.

Just one word of caution: Don't let other people hijack your need to talk by telling you their own stories. It's very common for well-meaning people to take in your news and rather than listening to you immediately grab the spotlight with their own story about their infected big toe last year at the beach. You are thinking, "How can they even compare something so minor to my breast cancer?" But before you know it, you are comforting them instead of the other way around.

As sociologist Dr. Jan Yager describes in her book *When Friendship Hurts: How to Deal With Friends Who Betray, Abandon, or Wound You,* "A close friend is one who listens closely without judging, who does not interrupt or recount her problems when you're telling her yours. She or he is 'unmistakably unselfish.' "

Pat Spicer helps out with her own follow-up question. "Have you always been the one who listened to how crazy her mother-in-law makes her every time the mother-in-law comes to dinner or what's wrong with Aunt Sally? If you've always been the giver in the relationship, you may find your relationship with this person isn't built on a real give-and-take dialogue."

Once you let the cat out of the bag with your news, there's no going back. One thing that happens to many women and their partners after a diagnosis of breast cancer is that their extended family and friends come to expect regular and frequent updates on your latest health news. As if you didn't have enough to do and worry about already!

Breast cancer husband Dave Balch explains, "There's no easy way to do this but it has to be done. The problem is once you start telling people then you start a chain reaction that ends up being tremendously stressful on you. There's a morbid curiosity. But on the other hand, a lot of people care about you and they want to know what's going on and they want to be included."

6. Will this person make things easier or harder for me once they know my news?

This is the "what's in it for me?" question. Let's face it. It's your diagnosis, your news, and your breast. You shouldn't feel obligated to tell toxic relatives, helicopter friends, or the people most likely to freak out.

Some people in your life will handle the news well and be very supportive of you, maybe even surprising you with their heartfelt generosity. People you may not feel especially close to may show you an outpouring of good cheer and practical assistance, like offering to drive you to your treatments. Others—sometimes the very people that you assumed you could count on—cope one hundred times worse than you ever could have imagined. They immediately run in the other direction as fast as they can, maybe never to be seen or heard from again. Unfortunately, sometimes "runners" include husbands, partners, and close family members or friends.

Other people may instantly morph into something as unpleasant as a critic ("What did you do to cause your breast cancer?"), a self-absorbed bubblehead ("I'm just glad that's not me with breast cancer!"), or perhaps give you the silent treatment, acting like you have leprosy instead of breast cancer. There is still a myth out there among some people that cancer is contagious; perhaps someone you know needs to be reassured that this isn't true. Just keep in mind

... cancer diagnosis from a close friend or family member is significantly more difficult than keeping a secret from the general public or acquaintances.

The people closest to you already know your habits and behaviors, and keeping a big secret may naturally raise their suspicions. Or perhaps you've never had a close relationship with your father and now you feel doubly burdened by that fact plus agonizing about telling him about your breast cancer.

Depending on who this person is to you, you might find that the secret of your diagnosis has taken over your relationship, causing a gaping distance between you. Also be prepared for some people to react unexpectedly. Mary Louise, sixty-nine, of Reno, Nevada, says with sadness, "Since my illness, some friends no longer contact me. I make them uncomfortable if I talk about my illness. I think they're just worried about their own boobs."

On the other hand, social worker Pat Spicer comments, "You may find the person who comes out of the woodwork, someone who might have been just a casual acquaintance and turns out to be the most wonderful support system."

8. Will telling this person about my diagnosis be an unfair burden to him or her?

Everyone has a lot going on. There may be some people who might not handle your news well, such as an elderly grandparent who is battling her own cancer. Perhaps you can be considerate by limiting specifics ("I've got an illness") or sharing your diagnosis with mutual friends or relatives first.

You may feel you don't want to bother some people or put them out. If you are worried about being a burden to others, consider:

- Most people probably do care and do want to help you.
- Letting others help may ease your burdens more than you initially anticipate.
- Would you be willing to help this person yourself if the tables were turned?

The key is not to assume automatically you'll tell everyone you can think of. Just spend a minute or two in their shoes first to make sure you won't somehow cause this person unnecessary grief.

9. What do I tell my employer? Am I obligated to tell? What about telling the others I know at my job?

When you are deciding about telling your employer, there are many considerations. These include the type of job you have, how much time off you'll need for your treatments, and whether or not you have health-insurance coverage through your employer. You may not have any choices about whether or not to tell your employer, but you can probably still control how and when you tell.

A diagnosis of breast cancer will test your relationship with your employer just as it will test your relationship with your partner. In both cases, if the relationship before you got breast cancer was a good one, chances are your cancer diagnosis will have a minimal impact. If you've had a previously stable and fairly happy employment situation, you may find great support from your employer and coworkers. Your coworkers may be among your closest friends, too. On the other hand, if you don't consider your employment sit-

ule earlier than my doctor had predicted."

Other breast cancer patients have less positive experiences in their workplaces when they first tell their news. Diane, fifty-three, a graphic designer in Rapid City, South Dakota, tells her story: "My employer gave me the time off I needed, but now I'm worried that I'll be the first one laid off next year. I had to tell my boss and the HR department, but wish I hadn't told anyone else. After I made the announcement in my office, people stared at my boobs like they were trying to see my illness through my clothes. One guy even asked me which one was 'in trouble.' "

With improved treatments, increasing survival rates for breast cancer, and supportive employment legislation, there's growing protection for cancer survivors on the job. In 2005, researchers at Pennsylvania State University found that although about 40 percent of women stopped working during their cancer treatment, most of them retuned to work during the first year following treatment. There's more about employment in chapter 16 on financial management.

10. How do I prefer to handle others' questions and reactions to my diagnosis?

This is again a matter of your personal preferences for communication and whom you decide to include in your "Tell" bucket. Just be aware that you'd be really, really smart to plan in advance how to handle the potential barrage of people who will want to be personally involved.

Breast cancer husband Dave Balch explains why. "It's very stressful to keep everyone up to date with progress reports. It takes a tremendous amount of time and is very tedious, repeating all the same stories over and over again." There's a wide range of options for coping with questions and reactions from your well-intentioned but sometimes clueless family and friends. For example, you can use humor to deflect negativity or melodramatic reactions, factual summaries to keep everyone well informed, or just have good crying jags with your loved ones. This question is just to help you consider that not only are you dealing with your own reactions to a diagnosis of cancer, you'll also be dealing with others' reactions as well.

There are also Web sites like CaringBridge.org where you can post information for supporters to read online.

❯ The Magic Question

Whom do I trust?

Trust is as important as it is illusive and complicated. It is a precious resource that can't be won overnight but can evaporate instantly even in the closest of relationships.

This question is potentially a deal breaker. Even the most fun, knowledgeable, convenient, important, or intimate people in your life may not pass the trust test. Not sure whom to trust? Here's another Magic Question to help you decide. Ask yourself, "Would I play poker with him or her over the phone?" If you answer yes, that's real trust!

Depending on how important privacy is to you, think in advance how much you might be bothered if your breast or health is the fodder for discussion behind your back. Once you get a clearer

work.

No matter how well you know them, some people will surprise you by being more positive or negative than you expected. Just as you've had your own unique way of handling your diagnosis, each person in your life is a unique individual and will react in his or her own way. Some newly diagnosed breast cancer patients feel the need to acknowledge publicly, share, and confront their cancer, choosing not to hide behind a false front of smiley faces. Others prefer to order up a supersize batch of smiley faces and find relief in not having to have anything but "have a nice day" type of conversations. There are no-one-size-fits-all rules, no rights, no wrongs, and no judgments here.

Over time you may find this whole issue has become a nonissue. Most important, do whatever it takes to reduce any extra stress in your life caused by your relationships. Instead, focus your time and energy on your healing process and seek the support of those who will be your best companions during your cancer journey to better health.

THE 10 BEST RESOURCES
American Cancer Society. "How Do I Talk to People About My Diagnosis?" www.cancer.org/docroot/ESN/content/ESN_2_1X_Sharing_a_cancer_diagnosis_with_family_and_friends.asp?sitearea=ESN.

American Cancer Society. "Talking About Cancer." www.cancer.org/docroot/ESN/esn_2.asp.

American Cancer Society. "Talking with Friends and Relatives About Your Cancer." www.cancer.org/docroot/ESN/content/ESN_2_1x_Com municating_with_Friends_and_Relatives_About_Your_Cancer.asp?site area=ESN.

Canadian Cancer Society. "Telling People about a Cancer Diagnosis." www.cancer.ca/ccs/internet/standard/0,3182,3172_369293_99086089 3_langId-en,00.html.

Carr, Kris. "Go Ahead—Use the Cancer Card," in *Crazy Sexy Cancer Tips*. Guilford, CT: Globe Pequot Press, 2007.

Imber-Black, Evan. *The Secret Life of Families: Making Decisions About Secrets: When Keeping Secrets Can Harm You, When Keeping Secrets Can Heal You—And How to Know the Difference.* New York: Bantam Press, 1999.

Livestrong (Lance Armstrong Foundation). "Telling Others You Are a Survivor: Suggestions." www.livestrong.org/site/c.khLXK1PxHmF/b.26 60785/k.4A1F/Telling_Others_You_are_a_Survivor_Suggestions.htm.

National Cancer Institute. "Sharing Your Feelings About Cancer." www .cancer.gov/cancertopics/takingtime/page4.

Neuharth, Dan. *Secrets You Keep from Yourself: How to Stop Sabotaging Your Happiness.* New York: St. Martin's Press, 2004.

Yager, Jan. *When Friendship Hurts: How to Deal With Friends Who Betray, Abandon, or Wound You.* New York: Fireside, 2002.

American author

Your diagnosis of breast cancer has a profound impact on your entire family. If you have children, not only do you have to cope with the factual and emotional overload this diagnosis brings you, but you are likely also to be very concerned about how and when to tell your children. No matter what their ages, telling your children that you have cancer is difficult.

The decision to tell your children is a deeply personal one with no hard-and-fast rules. You can talk it over with your partner/their father, other family members, friends, or professional counselors, but ultimately it's your decision. No matter what your children's ages, this is one more conversation on your cancer roller-coaster ride of emotions and fears that you never asked for or wanted. And you thought telling them about the birds and the bees was tough!

This chapter's list of 10 Best Questions will help you decide how and when to tell your children. It focuses on "the big talk," your initial explanation to your children of what you've learned about your diagnosis. Use the following Best Questions to ask yourself (*not* your children) prior to breaking your news. These questions will help you think through in advance about your upcoming big talk with your kids and to be better prepared for your actual conversation with them.

You'll need many more conversations and more question-and-answer sessions over the course of your treatments and recovery time, but these Best Questions will get you started. They will work for children of all ages from two through eighteen because these are questions to ask yourself, not your children.

The experts on children and cancer diagnoses all believe that honesty is the best policy when it comes to talking with your children. This honesty extends to telling them the full truth and using the word "cancer." The reasoning is that if your kids don't hear the scary word "cancer" from you, or if your diagnosis is kept from them as a terrible secret, once they finally do know, it will be a lot more horrifying for them than the truth ever could have been.

Advanced oncology nurse Melissa Craft explains the problem with keeping secrets using an analogy from the Harry Potter book series. She says, "Tell them now because they are going to know. Their imagination of what's wrong is actually going to be worse than the reality. It's like Harry Potter and Voldemort. If it's so bad that you're not even going to talk about it, not even use the word, you let cancer create a power that is beyond what it really should have."

In fact, CancerCare's social worker Win Boerckel believes you are only fooling yourself if you think your children won't know. He says, "If you tell them nothing, don't think that they know nothing. Children read you continuously every waking minute. They are constantly looking—not just listening to your words—to see what your expressions, body language, and energy levels are saying, too. They can tell when something is seriously wrong. No one is that good an actress."

The following Best Questions include suggestions for younger children as well as for teenagers. You know your children better than anyone else, so don't ignore your own instincts when planning this talk. You'll find your own best way to do this hard task. The Question Doctor sincerely hopes the following questions will help you feel less overwhelmed and more in control as you tell your children about your breast cancer.

>>> THE 10 BEST QUESTIONS
Before Telling Your Children About Your Breast Cancer

1. What is the best time and place to tell my children about my diagnosis?

There are two key considerations for answering this "when" and "where" question. First, you want to choose a place where you will be physically and emotionally comfortable. Second, you want to avoid outside distractions. The best place might just be your living room with the TV, video games, and cell phones turned off. Perhaps you have a favorite restaurant or park where you and your children have shared good times in the past.

If you think you or your children will cry, then a public place may not be a good idea. Ideally, you'll want some privacy and quiet. Chances are you and your partner already know your best answer to this question, so now figure out how to get everyone's focused attention. Kids of all ages have notoriously short attention spans.

2. Who else (if anyone) do I want to be there when I first break the news to my children?

There are many variables to consider as you try to line up the best surroundings, time, and people for breaking your news. For example, if your children have a biological father not currently living with you, you may want to include him during the discussion. Or perhaps you have other close family members who want to be there to support you, like your parents or your partner's parents. In another scenario, you may have older children who no longer live at home who you want to include in this conversation.

Another angle on this question is to include someone else who will be personally supportive of you, especially if you are dreading this conversation or feel overwhelmed by everything else going on. You may want to invite close family friends or the children's godparents. The only caveat is not to include others who may be emotionally unstable themselves during this conversation.

If you have more than one child, another consideration is whether or not you want to tell all your children at once or tell them separately. If you anticipate a wide range of reactions or if your children are far apart in age, separate sessions might be your best strategy. Again, there aren't any right or wrong answers or decisions, just worthy considerations to think about before talking with your children about your breast cancer.

3. What will be my children's most likely reactions to the news about my diagnosis?

Children have many different reactions when they learn their mom has cancer. They can be afraid, confused, guilty, or angry. If you have young kids, let them know that feelings are never wrong and whatever they are feeling is okay and normal. Tell them that you have feelings, too, and sometimes your feelings change from one day to the next, just like theirs.

Teenagers can be unpredictable and can have a wide range of possible reactions. Your son or daughter may feel embarrassed or uncomfortable because this cancer is in your breast. Many teens are immature about bodily functions and overly conscious of appearances. Your daughter may be worried about her own health and mortality. If you anticipate this reaction, you can be ready to ex-

plain your specific diagnosis along with the ~~~
inherited breast ~~~~~

...... ~~u can also practice
.... ahead of time either by yourself or with the children's father/your partner to boost your self-confidence. Look back to chapter 14 on dealing with emotions to help you consider the range of possible emotional responses to expect from your teen or adult children.

4. What factual information about breast cancer do I want to give my children?

It's very important that you give your children accurate information so they don't invent their own explanations, which are likely to be many times worse than reality. Use age-appropriate language and details to explain your disease. Don't be afraid to use the words "cancer" or "breast." Show or tell your children where your cancer is located. As you tell about your cancer, emphasize that you didn't cause it and they didn't cause it either.

There are many resources to help you put your diagnosis into age-appropriate words, including picture and activity books listed in the resource list at the end of this chapter and in the bibliography. Other helpful resources are oncology social workers, cancer support groups, and nurse navigators, all with a potential wealth of experience and guidance for you.

Some teens want highly detailed information about your diagnosis, treatment plan, and prognosis. If this will be true of your teenagers, be ready with a list of Web sites, books, or resources that they can look up on their own. This process of searching for Web sites might also give your teenager some personal space and privacy to absorb the news as well as a sense of being back in control of the situation.

By all means, be honest with your teenagers. Some teens are ultrasensitive about seeking and knowing the truth when adults are involved and could resent any information they feel is incomplete or inaccurate.

5. How can I best describe to my children my upcoming cancer treatment and how my treatment will affect their lives?

Explaining your cancer and treatments to children can be overwhelming, especially when this task calls up your own fears and uncertainties. But children need information to help them prepare for what is about to happen to you and how it will affect them.

If you have young children (ages two to eight), they don't need a lot of detailed information about your treatments. Older children (ages nine through teens) will want to know more and will be more inquisitive about your treatments. If you find this is a hard discussion—perhaps because of your own fears or lack of facts—consider using one of the picture or activity books for younger children in the resource list at the end of the chapter.

Prepare your children for any physical changes you might have during treatment, such as hair loss, extreme tiredness, or weight loss. Let them know that their needs will be taken care of while you are undergoing cancer treatments. Emphasize normalcy in the family's routines and how you (and your partner) will do everything possible to keep the children's lives from being affected by your treatment schedule. For example, "Dad will pick you up from softball practice instead of Mom for a while."

Be honest with your children that you may not feel well after treatments. Some oncologists suggest bringing your child along to a couple of office appointments or to tour the cancer care facility to take the scare factor out of your treat~~

check ~~

~~progress. For young children, let them know that you aren't leaving them. Tell them more than once that the treatments or surgery is the best way that the doctors have to make mommy well again.

6. How can I reassure my children about my cancer and calm their fears?

Reassure your children that they will be cared for no matter what. Tell them that even if you can't always provide their care directly in the upcoming weeks, their needs are important and you'll make alternative arrangements for their well-being.

Again, giving your kids specific examples that they can easily relate to will help them to better understand and trust you. Teenagers especially need to be reassured about consistency. For example, tell your teen that you or your partner will make sure they can still attend their normal activities and social events.

Explain to your young children that no matter how naughty they may have been these last few weeks, they are not the reason that you are sick. Show your kids a lot of love and affection, as always, and let them know that even though things are now different, your love for them hasn't changed. Also reassure them that they can't catch cancer like they can catch a cold and that just because you have cancer, that doesn't mean they will someday have it too.

Encourage your children to share their feelings with you, including ones that are uncomfortable or scary. Also let them know that it's okay to say, "I don't feel like talking right now." If you're afraid your children's fears on top of your own may be just too much overload, talk to your partner or another loved one before telling your kids and ask for their personal support.

7. Who else can my children talk to about my cancer and to get support?

Let your kids know it's okay if they want to turn to other people for support, comfort, and advice. You and your partner might personally feel more at ease if you don't shoulder this entire burden yourselves.

This preplanning session with Best Questions will give you a chance to figure out who in your children's lives is most likely to be an especially good outside support source and listening ear if your kids need one. As you run through the possibilities, be sensitive and put yourself in your children's shoes. Try to avoid suggesting someone they don't like or know well. For example, forget Aunt Marsha if you already know your kids think she's a jerk.

Your children's support system may include other relatives, friends, religious or community leaders, teachers, coaches, your medical team, professional counselors, or oncology social workers. Encourage your children to ask questions of these adults for factual information and to share their feelings.

Older children may benefit from joining an age-appropriate support group for peer reassurance and information about the upcoming changes in their lives. An example is the CancerCare for Kids® Program (www.cancercare.org). There are also peer-to-peer networks and online chat rooms for kids whose parents have cancer. With obvious minor adjustments, your teenager can use some of the Best Questions in chapter 15 on support groups to make his own decisions about joining one.

Some teenagers may treasure their privacy more than talking to outsiders. If this sounds like your teen, suggest support from a friend's parent or a member of your ~~~~ ~~~~ ~~~~

... matter what age they are. Give them age-appropriate tasks such as bringing you a glass of water or an extra blanket for younger children, or driving you to a doctor's appointment for your teenager with a new driver's license.

Marion, forty-four, who lives in Iron River, Michigan, shares her story: "When I came home from the hospital, I wanted to be in charge again but simply didn't have the energy. It was so hard to ask my family for help! I finally realized that when my kids offered to help me, it was because they wanted to contribute to my recovery."

Teens may be overly sensitive to how they are being treated while you are healing. Try to find tasks that are helpful yet send the message that you respect them as almost-adults. This can help them feel more in control about the effect of your illness on their own lives.

On the flip side, don't demand too much of your older children. Several studies have concluded that some lifelong insecurities start in the teen years when a parent is diagnosed with a life-threatening illness. The teenager is continually asked to take on more household duties or to care for younger siblings beyond normal expectations. This can lead to the teenager having major inner conflicts, holding long-term resentments, and his or her own health problems, such as severe depression.

9. What questions are my children likely to ask?

If you anticipate your children's questions in advance, it will give you time to prepare good answers. This preplanning step gives you more control and may ease your mind about having this big talk with your kids.

As you listen to their questions, make sure you fully understand their questions (including any unspoken emotions such as fear, anger, or resentment) and that they fully understand your answers. Take into account their ages and prior experiences with serious illnesses in your family. For example, they may still remember Grandpa's lung cancer, his passing, and his funeral. This old memory may be unnecessarily affecting how they are interpreting your news.

The most obvious question for most children, especially younger ones, is to ask you if you are going to die and then what will happen to them. Child experts say it's important *not* to tell your kids that you won't die, but rather to say you and your doctors are doing everything you can to make you well again.

One way to prepare is to go back to chapter 1 and questions about your initial diagnosis of breast cancer and find age-appropriate language to answer for your children the same questions you asked your doctor. These questions include the kind of breast cancer, its medical name, the tumor's location, size, and spread, your prognosis, and an overview of your treatment plan.

If you don't know the answer to some of your kids' questions, don't panic. Say, "I don't know. I'll try to find out the answer and let you know." For older children, you can refer them to books or Web sites to learn more on their own. Be prepared for your older daughter's fears about inherited breast cancer by being ready with the facts to give her and comforting words to ease her concerns.

10. What is the worst question my children could ask me? What are their worst possible reactions? How can I be prepared for this worst-case scenario?

In addition to questions about your death, what else could your children ask you? What's the very worst thing that could happen or be said during the "big tall"?

...... your justification for not telling your children. We've already established how important it is that you tell your children and that they hear about it first from you.

Another way of thinking about this question is to figure out what your children *won't* ask you. Depending on your children's ages and personalities, they may clam up and not say a word in response to your news or abruptly leave the room. This might be your worst-case scenario, since you won't know how much they understood or want to know.

Nubia, twelve, who lives near Philadelphia, remembers her initial reactions. "I was scared by my mother's cancer. She had always taken care of me and my little brother since my dad left. I was afraid I wouldn't be strong enough to help her through her recovery. I was afraid that she might not recover. I was afraid to talk about my fears with her because I didn't want to upset her."

Don't think of this "big talk" as an all-or-nothing deal. Your children will need to hear about your breast cancer in stages and over time, just like you've had to let it sink in slowly too.

❯ The Magic Question

What are my own biggest fears about my cancer diagnosis?

There's nothing wrong with expressing your fears and emotions to your children. In fact, they are likely to expect you to. But this Magic Question aims to help you be flat-out honest with yourself as you identify your very most personal Achilles' heel or areas of greatest fears. It's important to do this before you initiate this conversation with your children. Kids, even younger ones, instinctively know where your raw edges are and may take direct aim, either unconsciously or, with some teens, as a calculated response.

For example, teens and some younger children may automatically understand the significance of breast cancer to your intimate relationship with their father or your current partner. They may blurt out, "Is Dad going to leave us?" or "Are you going to continue sleeping together while you're sick?" On the surface, these are rather innocent questions, but they have the potential of stabbing you in the heart. Your children are openly expressing—saying out loud!—the very fears haunting you at night and the ones you feel least comfortable acknowledging or discussing. By asking yourself this Magic Question in advance, you'll be more composed and able to respond with a less emotionally overwrought answer.

CONCLUSION

When you are helping your kids cope with your diagnosis of breast cancer, it's impossible to be prepared for every situation or everything they might say. This is normal and OK. Coping with breast cancer may leave you feeling emotional and vulnerable, especially as you consider telling your kids and caring for them during your treatment. But it's important to tell them about your cancer in age-appropriate language that is honest and forthright, as well as including your children in your care during treatment and recovery.

Although breast cancer can be overwhelming and disruptive to your everyday life, you still know better than anyone else how to care for your children. Trust your instincts for how best to support your kids during this difficult time and seek additional help from your partner/their father or from a professional counselor if needed.

For You

American Cancer Society. "Helping Children When A Family Member Has Cancer: Dealing With Diagnosis." www.cancer.org/docroot/ESN/content/ESN_2_1x_Helping_Your_Child_Deal_with_a_Cancer_Diagnosis_in_the_Family.asp?sitearea=ESN.

American Cancer Society. "Helping Children When A Family Member Has Cancer: Dealing With Treatment." www.cancer.org/docroot/ESN/content/ESN_2_1x_Helping_Your_Child_Deal_with_a_Family_Members_Cancer_Treatment.asp?sitearea=ESN.

American Cancer Society. "Helping Children When A Family Member Has Cancer: Understanding Psychosocial Support Services." www.cancer.org/docroot/CRI/CRI_2_6x_understanding_psychosocial_support_services_7.asp.

CancerCare. "Fact Sheet: Helping Children Understand Cancer: Talking to Your Kids About Your Diagnosis." www.cancercare.org/pdf/fact_sheets/fs_children_en.pdf.

CancerCare. "Fact Sheet: Helping Teenagers When a Parent Has Cancer." www.cancercare.org/pdf/fact_sheets/fs_teenagers.pdf.

Harpham, Wendy S. *When a Parent Has Cancer: A Guide to Caring for Your Children.* New York: HarperCollins, 2001.

Heiny, Sue P., Joan F. Hermann, Katherine V. Bruss, and Joy L. Fincannon. *Cancer in the Family: Helping Children Cope with a Parent's Illness.* American Cancer Society, 2001.

McCue, Kathleen, and Ron Bonn. *How to Help Children Through a Parent's Serious Illness.* New York: St. Martin's Press, 1996.

National Cancer Institute. "Talking with Family and Friends," in "When Someone You Love Is Being Treated for Cancer." www.cancer.gov/cancer topics/When-Someone-You-Love-Is-Treated/page6#d1.

Van Dernoot, Peter, and Madelyn Case. *Helping Your Children Cope with Your Cancer: A Guide for Parents and Families* 2nd ed. Long Island City, NY: Hatherleigh Press, 2006.

For Your Children

Ackermann, Adrienne, and Abigail Ackermann. *Our Mom Has Cancer.* Atlanta: American Cancer Society, 2001. Ages 9–12.

American Cancer Society. *Because . . . Someone I Love Has Cancer: Kid's Activity Book.* Atlanta: American Cancer Society, 2002.

CancerCare. CancerCare for Kids program. www.cancercare.org/get_help/special_progs/cc_for_kids.php.

Frahm, Amelia. *Tickles Tabitha's Cancer-tankerous Mommy.* Hutchinson, MN: Nutcracker Publishing, 2001. Ages 4–8

Gillette Cancer Connection. "For Teens and Kids." www.gillettecancer connect.org/women/family_friends/for_kids.asp.

Kids Konnected. "Kids Helping Kids." www.kidskonnected.org/.

Kohlenberg, Sherry. *Sammy's Mommy Has Cancer.* Chicago: Gareth Stevens Publishers, 1994.

National Cancer Institute. "When Your Parent Has Cancer: A Guide for Teens." www.cancer.gov/cancertopics/When-Your-Parent-Has-Cancer-Guide-for-Teens/PDF.

Numeroff, Laura, Wendy Schlessel Harpham, and David M. McPhail. *The Hope Tree: Kids Talk About Breast Cancer.* New York: Simon & Schuster Children's Publishing, 2001. Picture book.

Winthrop, Elizabeth Mahony, and Betsy Lewin. *Promise.* New York: Clarion Books, 2000. Preschool.

When you have cancer, you have many reasons to be upset. Down days are to be expected. Don't pretend to be cheerful when you're not. This can keep you from getting the help you need. Be honest and talk about all your feelings, not just the cheerful ones.

Helen, seventy-one, a breast cancer survivor who lives in Wabasso Beach, Florida, says, "The advice of well-meaning friends to be positive, optimistic, and upbeat can also be a call for silence. Don't let them force you to put on a fake smile when that's the last thing you feel like doing."

On the other hand, humor is a power ally in your cancer battle. Over the past decades, studies have found that humor can reduce pain, aid the immune system, and keep the brain alert. The message is simple: humor is healing. The medicinal power of laughter can fight your fear and uncertainty and help to lighten your load on your cancer journey.

Cancer survivor Brenda Elsagher in Burnsville, Minnesota, turned her terrible cancer experience into a new career as a stand-up comedian and author. She says, "I needed to laugh in the midst of all this. I needed to laugh because it's my way of coping. I decided I was going to look for the funny side of my cancer."

In his pioneering 1979 book *Anatomy of an Illness as Perceived by the Patient,* Norman Cousins asserted that "laughter therapy" cured him from a supposedly irreversible disease. "Nothing is less funny than being flat on your back with all the bones in your spine and joints hurting," he wrote. Cousins started watching old Marx Brothers films and TV's *Candid Camera* classics while still in the hospital. He discovered that ten minutes of genuine belly laughter had an anesthetic effect that allowed him to get two hours of pain-free sleep.

Most breast cancer survivors find their sense of humor again and face cancer down with a healthy shot of laughter. The healing power of humor is the gateway to your other positive emotions.

The funniest stories come from how you look at things—the medicine of laughter is often right in front of you in the form of your well-meaning but clueless friends and family members. Think back to all the times since your initial cancer diagnosis that someone has said something to you that was well-intended but either was so off-track or crass that it was downright laughable.

The author has collected these awful questions from hundreds of breast cancer survivors. So welcome to "The Hall of Shame." The infamous "hall of shameful questions" holds the 10 Worst Questions that others have asked a breast cancer survivor according to breast cancer support groups, online chat rooms, and from interviews for this book. So, here's what *not* to ask, especially when you don't know what to say!

>>>THE 10 WORST QUESTIONS
to Ask a Breast Cancer Patient

1. Did I tell you about my aunt Sally who got breast cancer last year and who dropped dead less than two months later?

One of the most universally despised and most common Worst Questions involves telling a long shaggy-dog story about someone else's cancer, especially one with a tragic ending. Aunt Sally has nothing to do with anything

Veronica, age forty-nine, from Shipman Hill, Vermont, recalls, "I'd find myself cringing, waiting for the same two phrases every time: 'I know exactly how you feel' and 'This is what happened to me.' I couldn't get them to listen to *me.*"

2. What did you do to cause your cancer?

One of the most common misconceptions in our hyper health-conscious society is that somehow people cause or are responsible for their own cancers. This is simply not true. No one knows with 100-percent certainty what causes most kinds of cancer, including breast cancer. This Worst Question indicates a blame the victim mindset. Don't fall for it. It's not your fault.

3. How long did they give you to live?

This innocent question reflects the asker's ignorance of breast cancer statistics and the myth that all cancer diagnoses are automatic death sentences. Sometimes people just don't know what else to ask except to ask "time" questions—how long, how short, how often, etc.

4. Can you still wear a bra?

Oh, please! Is this a nosy and insensitive question or what? You have the Question Doctor's permission to come up with an equally inappropriate response.

5. What are you so worked up about?

This question usually comes from the same creep who tells you that he had a hernia operation last year and he's just fine, thanks. This awful question lacks any shred of sympathy, empathy, or understanding about what's involved with the complexities and hardships of breast cancer treatment.

It's the opposite of Worst Question 3. Instead of assuming a worst-case scenario, now the asker has unconsciously assumed a best-case scenario. The asker has also discredited your need to share the information or feelings that you might have been on the verge of talking about.

6. Should you be eating that?

Coming from the right person and with the right tone of voice, this is an OK question. It shows concern for your health. But if your overbearing mother asks you this question over and over again, you might be tempted to go into orbit, just to keep from strangling her. Or if Marathon Mary at work is commenting on the food on your cafeteria tray as you walk by her, you're probably silently hating yourself for telling her about your breast cancer while also hating Mary because she claims she's never eaten a potato chip in her life.

Want an answer to "Should you be eating that?" Try "Probably not without a glass of wine to go with it." So there!

7. How does your husband/partner feel about this? Is he still romantic with you?

Again, coming from the right person, this can be a kind and caring question. The asker's motivation behind this question may be purely good-hearted and an invitation to talk. But if asked in a prying, inquisitive manner or by someone you aren't close to, this can

that question if you had a different kind of cancer, like lung or stomach. Their response will probably reveal a lot about their real motivations.

8. How much did your breast weigh?

No kidding. Two breast cancer survivors who live hundreds of miles apart claim to have been asked this slightly sick and twisted question after their mastectomies.

9. Is that a wig? Can I see your bald head?

Maybe you're cool with this question and can whip off your wig as you look the other person straight in the eye and ask back, "Want to borrow my hair?" If not, any version of "no" also works here.

10. Weren't you thinking about getting a boob job anyway?

The asker has erroneously equated your breast reconstruction surgery with a "boob job," a breast implant surgery for cosmetic reasons. The reasons behind these two surgeries are as different as night and day. Another variation of this Worst Question is asking you about your "tummy tuck" after a flap reconstruction surgery, implying you only wanted a free tummy tuck. Come on! There are lots of easier ways to get gorgeous.

THE QUESTION DOCTOR SAYS:

Communication experts make the following suggestions for the friends and family members who are talking with a cancer patient. Avoid saying:

> I know just how you feel.

> You need to talk.

> I know just what you should do.

> I feel helpless.

> I don't know how you manage.

Do say:

> I'm sorry this has happened to you.

> If you ever feel like talking, I am here to listen.

> Please let me know what I can do to help.

> You are an inspiration.

> The Magic Question

What's for dinner?
Sigh. Sob. Scream. Laugh. Reply, "Takeout again, my dear."

CONCLUSION
In order not to be offended by any of these Worst Questions, ask yourself, "Are these folks trying to upset me or are they trying to comfort me?" Usually the answer is "trying to comfort."

So instead of angry thoughts like, "How can you possibly know what this is like for me?" focus on their sincerity in trying to be helpful. Then

BEST RESOURCES

American Cancer Society. "Suggestions for Talking with the Person with Cancer." www.cancer.org/docroot/ESN/content/ESN_2_1X_Suggestions_for_talking_with_the_person_with_cancer.asp?sitearea=ESN.

American Cancer Society. "Survivor Learns to Sprinkle Bad News With Laughter." www.cancer.org/docroot/ESN/content/ESN_2_1x_Survivor_Learns_to_Sprinkle_Bad_News_With_Laughter.asp?sitearea=ESN.

Association for Applied and Therapeutic Humor. "Humor Resource Archive." www.aath.org/archive.htm.

Breese, Kristine. *Cereal for Dinner: Strategies, Shortcuts, and Sanity for Moms Battling Illness.* New York: St. Martin's Griffin, 2004.

Burton, Scott. *A Life in Balance.* Detroit: Inconvenience Productions, 1997.

Cancer Club. "Laughter Is the Best Medicine!" www.cancerclub.com/.

Cousins, Norman. *Anatomy of an Illness.* New York: W.W. Norton, 1979.

God Help Me! A Cancer Survivor's Bookstore. "Laughter Bookshelf." www.godhelpme.com/laughter.htm.

Klein, Allen. "Humor and Healing Links." www.allenklein.com.

National Cancer Institute. "Talking with Family and Friends," in "When Someone You Love Is Being Treated for Cancer." www.cancer.gov/cancertopics/When-Someone-You-Love-Is-Treated/page6#d1.

...their private cancer war and they are the victors. For some women, it's been a long and painful journey; even for those with early breast cancer, it's often no less emotionally and spiritually traumatic. Cancer is cancer no matter what type or stage you have.

The second finish line you cross is the realization that even though you've won the big battle against breast cancer and been "saved," you still have a lifelong struggle ahead as you resume your "normal" life. For many women, everyday aches and pains strike fear in their hearts that the cancer has come back. They are on constant alert for first warning signs, as well as still coping with the physical aftermath of treatment side effects like lymphedema, cancer fatigue, hair loss, or long-term hormone therapy.

This second finish line and your return to normalcy can also bring feelings of being let down, lost, and depressed. Many breast cancer survivors tell how their partners, families, and friends stopped hovering, pampering, or even inquiring about them because they figured the cancer crisis was over. CancerCare's Pat Spicer speaks from her twenty years of counseling experience: "Others think it's over after the treatments, the chemo, the radiation all end, but for the woman it's not. She's still looking at her own mortality."

Depression and stress are commonplace. Mary, fifty-four, who lives near Boston, says, "I knew I was still sick, but my family thought I was cured. My sisters even forgot to ask me at Thanksgiving about my cancer. They just thought it was over. But I am still depressed and worry a lot about a recurrence."

The truth is that "breast cancer is never completely over," observes radiation oncologist and author Marisa C. Weiss, M.D. Good communication makes for good medicine. Just remember that you don't need to be a medical genius. All you need are the right questions. Even the world's most famous genius, Albert Einstein, believed in the power of questions. He once said in reply to an interviewer's query about how he was different from other people, "It's my ability to ask the right questions, clearly and cleanly."

The Question Doctor sincerely hopes this book and its 10 Best Questions will light the way for you and be a faithful companion during your cancer journey. The best solutions to breast cancer's physical, emotional, and spiritual challenges start with having the Best Questions.

Think of this book as an inspiration to develop a lifelong habit of asking your own best questions in all kinds of other circumstances, from buying a car, to choosing your son's school, to deciding whether or not to marry someone. The framework of the 10 Best Questions will work for many later decisions, choices, and relationships.

Knowledge is power. The Best Questions are your secret weapon in the script you need to take control of your health. Asking questions is so empowering, no matter what the circumstance. Enjoy being on the other side of breast cancer and living your life to its fullest—and full of questions.

we regret any omissions or errors on this resource list. Inclusion on this list does not imply endorsement by the publisher or the author. We defined "best resource" as the most practical and content-rich information available with an emphasis on question lists and free online access.

THE 10 VERY BEST OF THE BEST RESOURCES FOR BREAST CANCER

American Cancer Society. www.cancer.org. Find here a treasure trove of educational and helpful resources. Call 1-800-ACS-2345.

Breastcancer.org. www.breastcancer.org. This popular Web site is brimming with solid information on all breast cancer topics.

Cancerbackup. www.cancerbackup.org.uk. A UK Web site that emphasizes practical advice.

Healthfinder.gov. www.healthfinder.gov. Web site links for more than 1,500 health-related organizations and publications.

Link, John, et al. *The Breast Cancer Survival Manual: A Step-by-Step Guide for the Woman with Newly Diagnosed Breast Cancer,* 4th ed. New York: Henry Holt, 2007.

Love, Susan, Karen Lindsey, and Marcia Williams. *Dr. Susan Love's Breast Book,* 4th ed. Cambridge: Da Capo Press, 2005. The breast cancer bible.

Mayo Clinic. "Breast Cancer." www.mayoclinic.org/breast-cancer/.

National Cancer Institute. "Breast Cancer." www.cancer.gov/cancertopics/types/breast. This is the U.S. government's goldmine for comprehensive information on all aspects of breast cancer. Call 1-800-4-CANCER (1-800-422-6237).

Susan G. Komen for the Cure. cms.komen.org/komen/index.htm. This Web site offers strong grassroots support, patient advocacy, advice, latest research, and educational programs.

Weiss, Marisa, and Ellen Weiss. *Living Beyond Breast Cancer: A Survivor's Guide to When Treatment Ends and the Rest of Your Life Begins.* New York: Times Books, 1998.

CHAPTER RESOURCES

Chapter 1 — The 10 Best Questions About Your Initial Diagnosis of Breast Cancer

American Cancer Society. *Breast Cancer Clear and Simple: All Your Questions Answered.* Atlanta: American Cancer Society, 2007.

American Cancer Society. "Detailed Guide: Breast Cancer." www.cancer.org/doc root/CRI/CRI_2_3x.asp?dt=5.

American Cancer Society. *Informed Decisions: The Complete Book of Cancer Diagnosis, Treatment, and Recovery,* 2nd ed. Atlanta: American Cancer Society, 2001.

Babylon Breast Cancer Coalition. www.babylonbreastcancer.org.

Breastcancer.org. www.breastcancer.org.

Canadian Cancer Society. "Questions to Ask Your Healthcare Team." www.cancer .ca/vgn/images/portal/cit_86751114/38/15/1176414334Questionstoask-Tool.pdf.

Cancerbackup. "Breast Cancer Information Centre." www.cancerbackup.org.uk/ Cancertype/Breast.

Cancerbackup. "How Breast Cancer Is Diagnosed." www.cancerbackup.org.uk/ Cancertype/Breast/Causesdiagnosis/Diagnosis.

CancerGuide. "Understanding Cancer Types and Staging." cancerguide.org/basic .html.

Canfield, Jack, Mark Victor Hansen, Patty Aubrey, and Beverly Kirkhart. *Chicken Soup for the Surviving Soul: 101 Healing Stories About Those Who Have Survived Cancer.* Deerfield Beach, FL: Health Communications, 1996.

Dr. Susan Love Research Foundation. "Breast Cancer Overview." www.susan lovemd.com/breastcancer/.

EbscoHost online database. "Questions to Ask Your Doctor About Breast Cancer." web.ebscohost.com.proxymu.wrlc.org/ehost (subscription required).

Imaginis. "Breast Cancer in Men." www.imaginis.com/breasthealth/bemen.asp.

Mayo Clinic. "Cancer diagnosis? Advice for Dealing with What Comes Next." www.mayoclinic.com/health/cancerdiagnosis/HQ00379. Interview with cancer specialist Edward T. Creagan, M.D.

Miller, Kenneth D., ed. *Choices in Breast Cancer Treatment: Medical Specialists and Cancer Survivors Tell You What You Need to Know.* Baltimore: The Johns Hopkins University Press, 2008.

National Breast and Ovarian Cancer Centre (Australia). "A Guide for Women with Early Breast Cancer." www.nbocc.org.au/resources/documents/EBC_ earlyguide.pdf.

National Breast Cancer Foundation. "Advice to Women Newly Diagnosed with Breast Cancer." www.nationalbreastcancer.org/about-breast-cancer/breast-cancer-library.

National Cancer Institute. "Fact Sheet: Improving Methods for Breast Cancer Detection and Diagnosis."

Star, Talking to Your Doctor: 10 Questions to Ask Before a Mammography or Cancer Treatment," May 9, 1996.

Rollin, Betty, and Jules Feiffer: *Here's the Bright Side: Of Failure, Fear, Cancer, Divorce, and Other Bum Raps.* New York: Random House, 1997.

University of California, San Francisco. "Questions to Ask Your Doctor." cc.ucsf .edu/crc/hm_questions.html.

U.S. Department of Health and Human Services, Agency for Healthcare Research and Quality (AHRQ). "Be Prepared for Medical Appointments: Build Your Question List." www.ahrq.gov/qual/beprepared.pdf.

U.S. Department of Health and Human Services, Agency for Healthcare Research and Quality (AHRQ). "The Next Steps After Your Diagnosis: Finding Information and Support." www.ahrq.gov/consumer/diaginfo.pdf.

Y-ME National Breast Cancer Organization. "Every Woman's Guide to Breast Cancer." www.y-me.org/publications/generalpubs/every_womans_guide.pdf.

Chapter 2 — The 10 Best Questions to Find a Top Oncologist or Surgeon

Administrators in Medicine. docboard.org.

American College of Surgeons. www.facs.org.

American Medical Association. www.ama-assn.org.

Barrett, Stephen. "Physician Credentials: How Can I Check Them?" www.quack watch.org.

ChoiceTrust/HealthPlus. www.choicetrust.com.

Consumerist. "Consumerist Kit: Intro to Choosing a Doctor." consumerist.com.

Cuello, Leo. "Ask the Doctor: Never Hesitate to Ask a Physician about Surgery, His Techniques." *San Antonio Express-News,* July 21, 1997.

Docinfo. www.docinfo.org.

Ferraro, Susan. "Surgical Scenarios: Why Preparation Is So Critical Before You Go Under the Knife." *New York Daily News,* May 21, 2000.

Healthbolt. "The 10 Questions You Need to Ask Your Doctor Before Surgery." www.healthbolt.net/2007/01/08/the-10-questions-you-need-to-ask-your-doctor-before-surgery/.

Health care choices. healthcarechoices.org.

Koop, C. Everett. *Koop: The Memoirs of America's Family Doctor.* New York: Harper-Collins, 1993.

Leeds, Dorothy. *Smart Questions to Ask Your Doctor.* New York: Harper Paperbacks, 1992.

Manning, Phil R., and Lois DeBakey. "Reading: Keeping Current," in *Medicine: Preserving the Passion in the 21st Century*, 2nd ed. New York: Springer, 2003.

Maurer, Janet M. *How to Talk to Your Doctor: The Questions to Ask*, New York: Simon & Schuster, 1986.

National Breast Cancer Foundation. "A Good Doctor-Patient Relationship in Breast Cancer." nbcf.healthology.com/hybrid/hybrid-autodetect.aspx?focus_handle=breast-cancer-information&content_id=1767&brand_name=nbcf.

National Cancer Institute. "Fact Sheet: Sentinel Lymph Node Biopsy: Questions and Answers." www.cancer.gov/cancertopics/factsheet/therapy/sentinel-node-biopsy.

National Institute on Aging. "Talking with Your Doctor: A Guide for Older People." www.niapublications.org/pubs/talking/index.asp.

Nowroozi, Christine K. "How to Choose the Right Doctor." *Nation's Business*, September 1993.

O'Brien, Sharon. "10 Questions to Ask Your Doctor Before Accepting Medical Treatment." seniorliving.about.com/od/doctorshospitals/a/medicaltreatmen.htm

Shiel, William C., Jr. "Surgery Questions to Ask Your Surgeon." www.medicinenet.com/surgery_questions/article.htm.

Time, "Choosing a Doctor and a Hospital," April 24, 2006.

Tyberg, Theodore, and Kenneth Rothaus. *Hospital Smarts: The Insider's Survival Guide to Your Hospital, Your Doctor, the Nursing Staff—And Your Bill!*, New York: Hearst Books, 1995.

University of California Medical Center at Irvine. "FAQ Express: What to Ask Your Doctor." www.ucihealth.com.

U.S. Department of Health and Human Services, Agency for Healthcare Research and Quality (AHRQ). "Pocket Guide to Good Health for Adults." www.ahrq.gov/ppip/adguide/adguide.pdf.

U.S. Department of Health and Human Services, Agency for Healthcare Research and Quality (AHRQ). "Your Guide to Choosing Quality Health Care." www.ahrq.gov/consumer/qntool.htm.

WebMD. "10 Questions Before Cancer Surgery." www.webmd.com/-cancer/10-questions-before-surgery.

Weiss, Marisa, and Ellen Weiss. "You and Your Doctors," in *Living Beyond Breast*

Cancer: A Survivor's Guide to When Tr~~
New York: T~

~~g and Breast Cancer." www.cancerbackup.org.uk/
~~ncertype/Breast/Causesdiagnosis/HER2testing.

Doctor's Doctor. "Translating the Report." www.thedoctorsdoctor.com.

Fayed, Lisa. "Types of Breast Cancer." cancer.about.com/od/breastcancer/a/cancer types.htm.

Kneece, Judy C. "Understanding Your Pathology Report," in *Your Breast Cancer Treatment Handbook: Your Guide to Understanding the Disease, Treatment, Emotions, and Recovery from Breast Cancer*, 6th ed. North Charleston, SC: Educare Publishing, 2004.

Lab Tests Online. "Breast Cancer." www.labtestsonline.org/understanding/conditions/breast.html.

Link, John, James Waisman, and Cynthia Forstoff. *The Breast Cancer Survival Manual: A Step-by-Step Guide for the Woman with Newly Diagnosed Breast Cancer*, 4th ed. New York: Henry Holt, 2007.

Love, Susan, Karen Lindsey, and Marcia Williams. "Weighing the Options," in *Dr. Susan Love's Breast Book*, 4th ed. Cambridge: Da Capo Press, 2005.

Love, Susan, Karen Lindsey, and Marcia Williams. "What Kind of Cancer Is It?" in *Dr. Susan Love's Breast Book*, 4th ed. Cambridge: Da Capo Press, 2005.

Mayer, Musa. *Advanced Breast Cancer: A Guide to Living with Metastatic Disease*, 2nd ed. Sebastopol, CA: Patient Centered Guides, 1998.

Mayer, Musa. *After Breast Cancer: Answers to the Questions You Are Afraid to Ask*. Sebastopol, CA: Patient Centered Guides, 2003.

Mayo Clinic. "Breast Biopsy Identifies Suspicious Breast Tissue." www.mayoclinic.com/health/breast-biopsy.WO00111.

Miller, Kenneth D., ed. *Choices in Breast Cancer Treatment: Medical Specialists and Cancer Survivors Tell You What You Need to Know*. Baltimore: The Johns Hopkins University Press, 2008.

National Breast Cancer Foundation. "Be Active in Your Breast Cancer Treatment." www.nationalbreastcancer.org/about-breast-cancer/breast-cancer-library.

National Comprehensive Cancer Network. "Breast Cancer Treatment Guidelines for Patients." www.nccn.org/patients/patient_gls/_english/_breast/1_intro duction.asp#Decisions.

Oregon Health & Science University. "What Is a Pathology Report?" www.ohsu .edu.

Perkins C.I., et al. "Association Between Breast Cancer Laterality and Tumor Location: United States, 1994–1998." *Cancer Causes & Control* 15, no. 7 (2004).

Sarp, Séverine, et al. "Tumor Location of the Lower-Inner Quadrant Is Associated with an Impaired Survival for Women with Early-Stage Breast Cancer." *Annals of Surgical Oncology* 14:1031–1039 (2007).

Weiss, Marisa, and Ellen Weiss. "Part Three: Coping with Lingering Side Effects of Treatments," in *Living Beyond Breast Cancer: A Survivor's Guide to When Treatment Ends and the Rest of Your Life Begins*. New York: Times Books, 1998.

Wikipedia. "Breast Cancer." en.wikipedia.org/wiki/Breast_cancer.

Chapter 4 — The 10 Best Questions to Assess a Doctor or Surgeon After Your First Consultation

Clark, Elizabeth J., ed. *Teamwork: The Cancer Patient's Guide to Talking with Your Doctor*. National Coalition for Cancer Survivorship, 2002. www.cancer advocacy.org/resources/publications/teamwork.pdf.

eHow. "How to Select a Doctor." www.ehow.com/how_2117763_select-a-doctor .html.

Federation of State Medical Boards. www.fsmb.org.

Gawande, Atul. *Better: A Surgeon's Notes on Performance*. London and New York: Picador, 2008.

Groopman, Jerome. *How Doctors Think*. Boston: Houghton Mifflin, 2007.

HealthGrades. www.healthgrades.com.

Manning, Phil R., and Lois DeBakey. "Evidence-based Medicine," in *Medicine: Preserving the Passion in the 21st Century*, 2nd ed. New York: Springer, 2003.

Montgomery, Kathryn. *How Doctors Think: Clinical Judgment and the Practice of Medicine*. New York: Oxford University Press, 2005.

Nowroozi, Christine K. "How to Choose the Right Doctor." *Nation's Business*, September 1993.

Schwartz, Marti Ann. *Lessons Learned from Cancer: A Poignant and Sometimes Irreverent Look at Life's Lessons Learned*. Bloomington, IN: 1st Books Library, 2002.

Schwartz, Marti Ann. *Listen to Me, Doctor: Taking Charge of Your Own Health Care*. San Francisco, CA: MacAdam/Cage Publishing, 1995.

Timmermans, Stefan, and Marc Berg. *The Gold Standard: The Challenge of Evidence-Based Medicine*. Philadelphia: Temple University Press, 2003.

USA Today, "Physicians: How to Choose a Doctor," February 10, 1990.

Wolinsky, Howard. "What to Ask a New D̶o̶c̶...
1995.

... *ailures of American*
...*ng a Statistic.* New York: Berkley Trade,

Miller, Jim. "Savvy Senior: Second Opinion Can Buy Peace of Mind." *Charleston Gazette*, May 10, 2004.

Parker-Pope, Tara. "5 Questions to Ask if You Are Diagnosed with Cancer." *The Virginian-Pilot & The Ledger-Star*, January 24, 2005.

University of Rochester Medical Center. "Questions to Ask If Your Doctor Recommends Tests." www.stronghealth.com/questions/Tests.html.

U.S. News & World Report, "When and How to Challenge Your Doctor," May 10, 1993.

WikiHow. "How to Decide What to Do." www.wikihow.com/Decide-What-to-Do.

Chapter 6 — The 10 Best Questions Before Breast Surgery

American Surgical Association. "Getting Surgery Right." www.americansurgical. info/abstracts/2007/7.cgi.

Benaron, Lisa. "The Uncertainty Principle: When Patients Accept Their Uncertain Future, They Become More Attuned to Their Lives." *MAMM Magazine*, March–April 2007. www.mamm.com/highlights.php?&year=2007&qbacki d=4613ba653731a6a3_79665&qbacktitl=March%20/%20April%202007 &seq=4.

Breastcancer.org. "Surgery." www.breastcancer.org/treatment/surgery/index.jsp.

Cancerbackup. "Treating Breast Cancer with Surgery." www.cancerbackup.org .uk/Cancertype/Breast/Treatment/Surgery.

Ettinger, Alan B., and Deborah M. Weisbort. *The Essential Patient Handbook: Getting the Health Care You Need—From Doctors Who Know.* New York: Demos Medical Publishing, 2004.

Healthbolt. "The 10 Questions You Need to Ask Your Doctor Before Surgery." www.healthbolt.net/2007/01/08/the-10-questions-you-need-to-ask-your-doctor-before-surgery/.

Journal of Clinical Oncology (press release), "Cancer Advances: More Women Are Choosing Double Mastectomy Even When Breast Cancer Is Confined to a Single Breast." October 22, 2007.

Kind, Gabriel, M.D. "Breast Cancer: New Surgical Options for Breast Cancer Patients!" *Cancer Weekly*, October 30, 2007.

Mayo Clinic. "Mastectomy versus Lumpectomy Guide." www.mayoclinic.com/health/mastectomy-lumpectomy/BC99999.

National Breast and Ovarian Cancer Centre (Australia). "Breast Surgery." www.nbocc.org.au/hsd/surgery.php.

National Cancer Institute. "Fact Sheet: Sentinel Lymph Node Biopsy: Questions and Answers." www.cancer.gov/cancertopics/factsheet/therapy/sentinel-node-biopsy.

National Research Center for Women & Families. "Surgery Choices for Women with Early-Stage Breast Cancer." www.center4research.org/surgeryoptions.html.

Obgyn.net. "Twenty Questions to Ask Your Surgeon: How to Know if You Are Getting Good Advice About Breast Disease and Breast Cancer." www.obgyn.net/displayarticle.asp?page=/bh/articles/twenty_questions.

OncologyChannel. "Mastectomy: Overview: Types." www.oncologychannel.com/mastectomy/index.shtml.

Ricks, Delthia. "Issues: What Gets Left Behind." *MAMM Magazine*, July–August 2006. www.mamm.com/highlights.php?&year=2006&qbackid=44be4438e91ca625_59676.

Smith, Amber. "Considering Surgery." *The Post-Standard* (Syracuse, NY), October 4, 2005.

Stanford University. "Breast Cancer Surgery." cancer.stanfordhospital.com/forPatients/services/surgery/breast/default.

Susan G. Komen for the Cure. "Questions to Ask the Doctor." www.komen.org.

Susan G. Komen for the Cure. "Surgical Treatment of Breast Cancer." cms.komen.org/stellent/groups/public/documents/komen_document/treatlocalsurgery.pdf.

U.S. Department of Health and Human Services, Agency for Healthcare Research and Quality (AHRQ). "Quick Tips—When Planning for Surgery." www.ahrq.gov/consumer/quicktips/tipsurgery.htm.

Chapter 7 — The 10 Best Questions for Choosing a Hospital

American Hospital Association. "Consumer Health Care Information"—comprehensive links list. www.aha.org/aha_app/resource-center/links/consumer-links.jsp.

American Hospital Association. "Patient Care Partnership: Understanding Expec-

tations, Rights and Responsibilities." ⸻
pcp_english_030730 ⸻ ¹⸻

Ameri⸻

⸻ice.shtml.

⸻ook: *A Guide to Becoming a Patient Advocate* ⸻. St. Paul: Llewellyn Publications, 2007.

⸻usiness *Wire*, "How to Choose a Hospital: Guidelines Issued by HealthGrades," May 28, 2003.

CalHospitalCompare.org. "Hospital Checklist." www.calhospitalcompare.org/Resources-and-Tools/Choosing-a-Hospital/Hospital-Checklist.aspx.

Cohn, Victor. "What Patients Should Ask." *Washington Post*, May 28, 1991.

Comarow, Avery. "Finding the Right Hospital for You: A Step-by-Step Guide to Getting the Best Care When You Have to Have It." *U.S. News and World Report*, July 19, 1999.

Consumer Reports. "Consumer Reports 2001 Annual Questionnaire on Patient Satisfaction." www.consumerreports.org (subscription required).

Consumer Reports. "Drug-resistant Bug Raises New Concerns," July 2007. www.consumerreports.org.

Elash, Anita. "The Hospital Patient's Action Plan." *Chatelaine*, August 1998.

Health Care Financing Administration and the Agency for Healthcare Research and Quality. *Choosing a Hospital: A Guide for People with Medicare*. Publication Number HCFA-10181 (2000). www.medicare.gov.

HealthGrades. "Hospital Report Cards." www.healthgrades.com.

Hospitalselect.com. "Consumer Reviews." www.hospitalselect.com.

Hutchinson, Roz. "Nursing Group Offers Questions that Reveal Care Level." *Wichita Business Journal*, April 5, 1996.

Jet. "Expert Urges Patients to Ask Questions to Prevent Errors During a Hospital Stay," September 11, 2000.

Joint Commission. "How to Prevent Medical Mistakes." www.jointcommission.org.

Kansas City Star, "Hospital Patients Need to Be Watchdogs, Too," July 23, 2006.

Kolata, Gina. "Looking for Answers When Choosing Care." *New York Times*, July 2, 2006.

National Patient Safety Foundation. "Safety as You Go from Hospital to Home." www.npsf.org/download/SafetyAsYouGo.pdf.

Newsweek, "Health: Hospital Hygiene Tip Sheet," May 21, 2007.

New York Times, "Surviving the Healing During a Hospital Stay," February 17, 2004.

Palm Beach Post, "Keep Eyes Open in Judging Whether a Hospital Is Safe," December 2, 2005.

PatientProtect.com. "To Choose Your Hospital or Your Private Clinic." www .patientprotect.com/en/hopital.html.

Reuters, Alert Net. "Want to Stop Disease from Spreading? Open a Window," February 26, 2007.

Sharon, Thomas A. *Protect Yourself in the Hospital: Insider Tips for Avoiding Hospital Mistakes for Yourself or Someone You Love.* Chicago: Contemporary Books, 2004.

Simon, Nissa. "Good Medicine: Hospitals Make Mistakes. What to Ask When Taking Charge of Your Treatment." *Time* magazine bonus section, August 16, 2004.

South Florida Sun-Sentinel, "How to Choose a Hospital," August 19, 2007.

University of Kansas Hospital (press release). "Six Important Things to Know About Preventing Hospital Infections. Infection Control Professional Offers Patient Tips to Guard Against Hospital Infections," April 2, 2007.

U.S. Department of Health and Human Services, Agency for Healthcare Research and Quality (AHRQ). "20 Tips to Help Prevent Medical Errors: Patient Fact Sheet." www.ahrq.gov/consumer/20tips.htm.

U.S. Department of Health and Human Services, Agency for Healthcare Research and Quality (AHRQ). "Choosing a Hospital." www.ahrq.gov/consumer/ qntascii/qnthosp.htm.

U.S. News/American Hospital Association. "Hospital Directory Search." www .usnews.com/usnews/health/hospitals/articles/mistakes.htm.

Van Kanegan, Gail, and Michael Boyette. *How to Survive Your Hospital Stay: The Complete Guide to Getting the Care You Need—And Avoiding Problems You Don't Need.* New York: Lynn Sonberg Books, 2003.

WebMD. "Work in Partnership with Your Health Professional to Prevent Medical Errors: Prevent Medical Errors During Hospital Stays." www.webmd .com/a-to-z-guides/work-in-partnership-with-your-health-professional-to-prevent-medical-errors-prevent-medical-errors.

West Suffolk Hospital (UK). "What To Ask Your Care Team Whilst In Hospital." www.wsh.nhs.uk/pals/PatInfo/redirect.aspx?ID=380.

Wikipedia. "Medical Errors." en.wikipedia.org/wiki/Medical_errors.

Chapter 8 — The 10 Best Questions About Chemotherapy

Adelphi NY Statewide Breast Cancer Hotline and Support Program. "Questions to Ask . . . About Breast Cancer: About Chemotherapy." www.adelphi.edu/ nysbreastcancer/questions.chemo.html.

Bruning, Nancy. *Coping with Chemotherapy: Comb~~~~*
  Information from a Chemo~~~
  ing C~~~

  . . . . www.chemocare.com/whatis/.
  . . . ~~~ Chemotherapy and Radiation Therapy, 4th ed. New York:
  McGraw-Hill, 2004.

Fayed, Lisa. "Chemotherapy Side Effects." cancer.about.com/od/chemotherapy/a/
  chemoeffects.htm.

Love, Susan, Karen Lindsey, and Marcia Williams. "Appendix A: Drugs Used for
  Systemic Treatment of Breast Cancer," in *Dr. Susan Love's Breast Book*, 4th ed.
  Cambridge: Da Capo Press, 2005.

Love, Susan, Karen Lindsey, and Marcia Williams. "Chemotherapy," in *Dr. Susan
  Love's Breast Book*, 4th ed. Cambridge: Da Capo Press, 2005.

M. D. Anderson Cancer Center, The University of Texas. "Chemotherapy." www
  .mdanderson.org/patients_public/about_cancer/display.cfm?id=DC30F674-
  7545-11D4-AEC300508BDCCE3A&method=displayFull.

Mooney, Michael. "The MAMM Guide to Chemotherapy." *MAMM Magazine.*
  July–August 2006. www.mamm.com/highlights.php?&year=2006&qbackid
  =44be4438e91ca625_59676&qbacktitl=July/August%202006&seq=2.

Murphy, Kevin. "Adjuvant Chemotherapy." cancerguide.org/adjuvant.html.

National Breast and Ovarian Cancer Centre (Australia). "Chemotherapy." www
  .breasthealth.com.au/treatment/chemotherapy.html.

National Cancer Institute. "Pain Control: A Guide for People with Cancer and
  Their Families." www.cancer.gov/cancertopics/paincontrol.pdf.

National Lymphedema Network. "Information for Patients." www.lymphnet.org/
  patients/patients.htm.

Oncologychannel. "Breast Cancer: Treatment, Prognosis and Prevention." www
  .oncologychannel.com/breastcancer/treatment.shtml.

Orndorff, Beverly. "Questions to Ask about Chemotherapy." *Richmond Times-
  Dispatch*, April 25, 1996.

Susan G. Komen for the Cure. "Chemotherapy." cms.komen.org/komen/About
  BreastCancer/Treatment/s_002828?ssSourceNodeId=298&ssSourceSiteId=
  Komen.

Wikipedia. "Chemotherapy." en.wikipedia.org/wiki/Chemotherapy.

Chapter 9 — The 10 Best Questions About Radiation Therapy

Academic Clinical Oncology and Radiology Research Network. "Patient Information." www.acorrn.org/Patient-Information.aspx.

American Cancer Society. "Radiation Therapy Effects." www.cancer.org/docroot/MBC/MBC_2x_RadiationEffects.asp?sitearea=MBC.

American College of Radiology. "Quality and Patient Safety." www.acr.org/SecondaryMainMenuCategories/quality_safety.aspx.

Augusta Chronicle, "Breast Cancer Radiation Therapy Increases Survival," January 21, 2004.

Cancerbackup. "Treating Breast Cancer with Radiotherapy." www.cancerbackup.org.uk/Cancertype/Breast/Treatment/Radiotherapy.

Cancer Treatment Centers of America. "Radiation Therapy." www.cancercenter.com/conventional-cancer-treatment/radiation-therapy.cfm.

Cancer Weekly, "Breast Cancer Therapy: Scientists at British Columbia Cancer Agency Discuss Research in Breast Cancer Therapy," November 6, 2007.

Heart Disease Weekly, "Breast Cancer, Radiation for Breast Cancer Not Likely to Increase Heart Attack Risk," May 27, 2007.

Kornmehl, Carol. *The Best News About Radiation Therapy: Everything You Need to Know About Your Treatment.* New York: M. Evans and Company, 2004.

Lyss, Alan P., Humberto Fagundes, and Patricia Corrigan. *Chemotherapy and Radiation For Dummies.* Hoboken, NJ: Wiley, 2005.

Mayo Clinic. "Radiation Therapy—Treatment Options." www.mayoclinic.org/radiation-therapy.

McKay, Judith, and Nanceé Hirano. *The Chemotherapy & Radiation Therapy Survival Guide*, 2nd ed. Oakland, CA: New Harbinger Publications, 1998.

Medicine.net. "Radiation Therapy." www.medicinenet.com/radiation_therapy/article.htm.

National Breast and Ovarian Cancer Centre (Australia). "Radiotherapy." www.breasthealth.com.au/treatment/radiotherapy.html.

National Lymphedema Network. "Information for Patients." www.lymphnet.org/patients/patients.htm.

O'Leary, Cathy. "Extra Radiation Tip for Younger Breast Cancer Patients." *The West Australian,* November 3, 2007.

Radiological Society of North America. "RSNA Education Portal: Breast Imaging." www.rsna.org/Education/archive/breast.cfm.

Susan G. Komen for the Cure. "Radiation Therapy." cms.komen.org/komen/AboutBreastCancer/Treatment/s_002823?ssSourceNodeId=298&ssSourceSiteId=Komen.

Y-ME National Breast Cancer Organization. "Partial Breast Irradiation (PBI): A

Shorter Path to Breast Cancer Radiation Th~~ ~~
tions/generalpubs/n~~~~~ ~~

~~…~~~~onaltherapies.~~

~~…~~ ~~…~~erapy Is." www.cancerhelp.org.uk/help/default
~~…p. page~~=24253#breast.

National Breast and Ovarian Cancer Centre (Australia). "Hormonal Therapies."
www.breasthealth.com.au/treatment/hormonetherapy.html.

Stephan, Pam. "Tamoxifen—Hormone Therapy to Prevent Breast Cancer Recurrence." breastcancer.about.com/od/treatments/p/tamoxifen.htm.

UpToDate. "Cancer." patients.uptodate.com/toc.asp?toc=cancer&title=Cancer.

WebMD. "Breast Cancer: Hormone Therapy Overview." www.webmd.com/breast-cancer/hormone-therapy-overview.

Chapter 11 — The 10 Best Questions Before Participating in a Clinical Trial

American Cancer Society. "Questions to Ask Your Doctor about Clinical Trials."
www.cancer.org/docroot/NWS/content/NWS_1_1x_Questions_to_Ask_Your_Doctor_about_Clinical_Trials.asp.

American College of Radiology Imaging Network. "Clinical Trials: How to Participate." www.acrin.org/PATIENTS/HOWTOPARTICIPATE/tabid/107/Default.aspx.

Baylor College of Medicine. "Research Study—Questions to Ask." www.bcm.edu/clinicalstudies/questions.cfm.

Canadian Cancer Society. "Questions to Ask About Clinical Trials." www.cancer.ca/ccs/internet/standard/0,3182,3172_367616_259329_langId-en,00.html.

Cichocki, Mark. "Top 10 Questions to Ask About Clinical Trials." aids.about.com/od/clinicaltrials/tp/trialq.htm.

Cohn, Victor. "The Patient's Advocate: Questions to Ask Before You Sign Up."
Washington Post, July 21, 1987.

Fayed, Lisa. "Cancer Clinical Trials." cancer.about.com/od/treatmentoptions/a/clinicaltrials.htm.

Friend, Tim. "Ask Your Doctor Questions." *USA Today*, September 13, 1995.

Greene, Kelly. "Playing Guinea Pig: More Clinical Trials Need Older Volunteers:
Should You Raise Your Hand?" *Wall Street Journal*, August 11, 2003.

Healthcare PR & Marketing News, "Questions To Ask During Clinical Trials," November 23, 2000.

International Federation of Pharmaceutical Manufacturers & Associations. "Clinical Trials Portal." clinicaltrials.ifpma.org/no_cache/en/myportal/index.htm.

Kalb, Claudia. "To Be a Guinea Pig: How to Decide on Entering a Clinical Drug Research Trial." *Newsweek*, October 19, 1998.

Keim, Brandon. "So You Want to Be a Gene Therapy Guinea Pig?" *Wired Science* blog, July 25, 2007. blog.wired.com/wiredscience/2007/07/so-you-want-to-.html.

Love, Susan, Karen Lindsey, and Marcia Williams. "Treatment Options: Local Therapy," in *Dr. Susan Love's Breast Book*, 4th ed. Cambridge: Da Capo Press, 2005.

MerckSource. "What Participants Need to Know About Clinical Trials." www.mercksource.com/pp/us/cns/cns_merckmanual_frameset.jsp?pg=http://www.merck.com/mmhe/sec25/ch307666/ch307666c.html.

National Breast and Ovarian Cancer Centre (Australia). "Clinical Trials." www.breasthealth.com.au/treatment/clinicaltrials.html.

National Cancer Institute. "Fact Sheet: Clinical Trials: Questions and Answers." www.cancer.gov/cancertopics/factsheet/Information/clinical-trials.

National Surgical Adjuvant Breast and Bowel Project. "NSABP Clinical Trials Overview." www.nsabp.pitt.edu/NSABP_Protocols.asp.

OncoLink. "Make Treatment Decisions with Cancer NexProfiler Tools." www.oncolink.upenn.edu/treatment/article.cfm?c=7&s=78&id=235.

Pesmen, Curtis. "Does It Pay to Be a Human Guinea Pig?" *Money Magazine*, May 2006.

Rayl, A.J.S. "The Complete Guide to Clinical Trials, Parts 1 & 2." *MAMM Magazine*, November–December 2005. www.mamm.com.

Susan G. Komen for the Cure. "Participating in Clinical Trials." cms.komen.org/komen/AboutBreastCancer/Treatments/s_002756?ssSourceNodeId=298&ssSourceSiteId=Komen.

Toronto Star, "Questions a Patient Should Ask the Doctor," August 24, 1987.

Wikipedia. "Clinical Trials." en.wikipedia.org/wiki/Clinical_trial.

Windsor Regional Cancer Centre. "Participating in a Trial: Questions to Ask Your Doctor." www.wrcc.on.ca.

Work & Family Life, "Is a Clinical Trial Right for Your Older Relative?" May 2003.

Y-ME National Breast Cancer Organization. "Discover Your Options: Is a Clinical Trial Right for You?" www.y-me.org/publications/generalpubs/Is_Clinical_Trial_Right_For_You.pdf.

Chapter 12—The 10 Best Questions f..

American Instir...

...omp_med/

... oafety and Effectiveness in Complementary Tech-
...ww.breastcancer.org/treatment/comp_med/safety.jsp.

Canadian Cancer Society. "Questions to Ask About Complementary and Alternative Therapies." www.cancer.ca/ccs/internet/standard/0,3182,3172_429199_451446262_langId-en,00.html.

Cassileth, Barrie, Gary Deng, Andrew Vickers, and K. Simon Yeung. *PDQ Integrative Oncology: Complementary Therapies in Cancer Care.* Ontario: BC Decker, 2005.

Collinge, William. *The American Holistic Health Association Complete Guide to Alternative Medicine.* New York: Grand Central Publishing, 1997.

Hay, Louise. *Heal Your Body.* Carlsbad, CA: Hay House, 1984.

Imaginis. "Alternative/Complementary Medicine." www.imaginis.com/breast health/alternative_print.asp.

Kabat-Zinn, Jon. *Wherever You Go, There You Are: Mindfulness Meditation in Everyday Life,* 10th ed. New York: Hyperion, 2005.

Lerner, Michael. *Choices in Healing: Integrating the Best of Conventional and Complementary Approaches to Cancer.* Cambridge, MA: MIT Press, 2006.

Love, Susan, Karen Lindsey, and Marcia Williams. "Complementary and Alternative Therapies," in *Dr. Susan Love's Breast Book,* 4th ed. Cambridge: Da Capo Press, 2005.

Mackenzie, Elizabeth R., and Birgit Rakel. *Complementary and Alternative Medicine for Older Adults: Holistic Approaches to Healthy Aging.* New York: Springer, 2006.

M. D. Anderson Cancer Centre. "Complementary/Integrative Medicine Education Resources." www.mdanderson.org/departments/CIMER/.

Memorial Sloan-Kettering Cancer Center. "About Herbs, Botanicals and Other Products." www.MSKCC.org/AboutHerbs.

National Cancer Institute. "Thinking about Complementary and Alternative Medicine." www.cancer.gov/cancertopics/thinking-about-CAM.

Park, Robert L. *Voodoo Science: The Road from Foolishness to Fraud*. London: Oxford University Press, 2001.

Siegel, Bernie S. *Love, Medicine and Miracles: Lessons Learned about Self-Healing from a Surgeon's Experience with Exceptional Patients*. New York: Harper Paperbacks, 1996.

Silverstein, Daniel D., and Allen D. Spiegel. "Are Physicians Aware of the Risks of Alternative Medicine?" *Journal of Community Health*, June 2001.

Spencer, John W., and Joseph J. Jacobs. *Complementary and Alternative Medicine: An Evidence-Based Approach*, 2nd ed. Oxford: Mosby, 2003.

Susan G. Komen for the Cure. "Complementary Therapies." cms.komen.org/komen/AboutBreastCancer/ComplementaryTherapies/index.htm.

Utilization Review Accreditation Council. "Consumer Resource Center." www.urac.org/consumers/resources/.

Weil, Andrew. *Healthy Aging: A Lifelong Guide to Your Physical and Spiritual Well-Being*. New York: Alfred A. Knopf, 2005.

Weil, Andrew. *Natural Health, Natural Medicine: The Complete Guide to Wellness and Self-Care for Optimum Health*, revised ed. Boston: Houghton Mifflin, 2004.

Wooddell, Margaret, and David Hess. *Women Confront Cancer: Twenty-One Leaders Making Medical History by Choosing Alternative and Complementary Therapies*. New York: NYU Press, 1998.

Chapter 13 — The 10 Best Questions About Breast Reconstruction Surgery

Breast Implants. "Breast Implants." www.breastimplants.com/breast_implants.htm.

Breastcancer.org. "Reconstruction." www.breastcancer.org/tips/reconstruction/index.jsp.

Canadian Society of Plastic Surgeons. "Breast Reconstruction." www.plasticsurgery.ca.

Cancerbackup. "Breast Reconstruction." www.cancerbackup.org.uk/Treatments/Surgery/Breastreconstruction.

Cancer Weekly, "Breast Cancer: New Surgical Options for Breast Cancer Patients," October 30, 2007.

Department of Health & Ageing, Therapeutic Goods Administration (Australia). "Breast Implant Information Booklet." www.tga.gov.au/docs/html/breasti.htm.

Grigg, Martha, et al., eds. "Information for Women about the Safety of Silicone Breast Implants." National Academies Press, 2000. www.nap.edu/catalog/9618.html.

Keller, Alex, M. D. "DIEP Flap Breast Reconstruction." www.breastflap.com.

MedicineNet. "Breast Reconstruction." www.m~d~ ·
struction/article.htm.

MedlinePlus "D

.. ~iki/Breast_implants.

..~uction." en.wikipedia.org/wiki/Breast_reconstruc

Chapter 14 — The 10 Best Questions to Maintain Your Emotional Health

American Cancer Society. "Tips for Coping with Breast Cancer." www.cancer.org/docroot/SPC/content/SPC_1_Tips_for_Coping_With_Breast_Cancer.asp.

American Psychological Association. "Breast Cancer Patients Who Actively Express Their Emotions Do Better Emotionally and Physically, Says New Study." www.apa.org/releases/canceremotion.html.

Beazley, Hamilton. *No Regrets: A Ten-Step Program for Living in the Present and Leaving the Past Behind.* New York: Wiley, 2004.

Benson, Herbert, and Miriam Z. Klipper. *The Relaxation Response.* New York: Harper Paperbacks, 2000.

Breastcancer.org. "Emotional Effects: Lymphedema." www.breastcancer.org/search.jsp?searchagain=emotions.

Canadian Breast Cancer Foundation. "Living with Breast Cancer: Emotions." www.cbcf.org/breastcancer/bc_livingbc_em.html.

Cancerbackup. "Feeling, Personality and Cancer." www.cancerbackup.org.uk/Treatments/Complementarytherapies/Generalinformation/Feelingspersonalityandcancer.

Cancerbackup. "The Emotional Effects of Cancer." www.cancerbackup.org.uk/Resourcessupport/Relationshipscommunication/Emotionaleffects.

Cancer Supportive Care Programs. "You're Not Alone: A Practical Guide for Maintaining Your Quality of Life While Living with Cancer." www.cancersupportivecare.com/Yana/support.html.

CancerSymptoms.org. "Depression: Key Points/Overview." www.cancersymptoms.org/depression/key.shtml.

Carr, Kris. "Holy Shit! I Have Cancer. Now What?" in *Crazy Sexy Cancer Tips.* Guilford, CT: Globe Pequot Press, 2007.

Granet, Roger. *Surviving Cancer Emotionally: Learning How to Heal*. New York: Wiley, 2001.

Harary, Keith. "The Stress Connection." *MAMM Magazine*, November–December 2005. www.mamm.com/pubs/MAMM/2005/11/01/110385?&p61–82.

Harpham, Wendy. *Diagnosis: Cancer: Your Guide to the First Months of Healthy Survivorship*, revised ed. New York: W. W. Norton, 2003.

King, Judith. *Breast Cancer Answers: Practical Tips and Personal Advice From A Survivor*. Franklin Lakes, NJ: New Page Books, 2004.

Kirkhart, Beverly. *My Healing Companion*. Santa Barbara, CA: Comeback Press, 2001.

Kübler-Ross, Elisabeth. *On Death and Dying*. New York: Macmillan, 1969.

Kübler-Ross, Elisabeth. *On Grief and Grieving: Finding the Meaning of Grief Through the Five Stages of Loss*. New York: Simon & Schuster, 2005.

Living Beyond Breast Cancer. "Women Discuss Emotions After Breast Cancer." www.lbbc.org/content/news/women-discuss-emotions-after-breast-cancer.asp?section_tag=G.

National Coalition for Cancer Survivorship. "Cancer Survival Toolbox." www.canceradvocacy.org/toolbox/.

Ovitz, Lori M. *Facing the Mirror with Cancer: A Guide to Using Makeup to Make a Difference*. Chicago: Belle Press, 2004.

Piver, Susan. *How Not to Be Afraid of Your Own Life: Opening Your Heart to Confidence, Intimacy, and Joy*. New York: St. Martin's Press, 2007.

Stamberg, Susan. *Talk: NPR's Susan Stamberg Considers All Things*. New York: Random House, 1993.

Stephan, Pam. "Emotional Stages of Breast Cancer During Diagnosis, Treatment and Survival." breastcancer.about.com/od/lifeduringtreatment/ss/emotion_stages.htm.

Stephan, Pam. "Emotions and Breast Cancer: Expressing, Coping, Surviving." breastcancer.about.com/od/diagnosis/a/emotions_coping.htm.

Chapter 15 — The 10 Best Questions
Before Joining a Support Group

African American Breast Cancer Alliance. Online support group. www.aabcainc.org.

American Cancer Society. "Considerations When Looking for a Support Group." www.cancer.org/docroot/ESN/content/ESN_1_1X_Considerations_when_looking_for_a_support_group.asp?sitearea=&level=.

American Cancer Society. "Reach to Recovery" (national and local discussion groups). www.cancer.org/docroot/ESN/content/ESN_3_1x_Reach_to_Recovery_5.asp?sitearea=ESN.

Breast Cancer Group. "Welcome to the Breast C~~~~ ~
group.org.

~~~~~~~~. ~~oups." cancer
~~~~~~~~~~groups.htm.

~~~~ng Our Risk of Cancer Empowered. Online community for women with increased risk of cancer. www.facingourrisk.org.

Gilda's Club Worldwide. "Find a Clubhouse." www.gildasclub.org/findaclub house.asp.

HER2support.org. Online support group for women with the HER2/neu gene. www.HER2support.org.

IBC Support. Online support group for women with inflammatory breast cancer. www.ibcsupport.org.

Lesbians & Cancer. "Support and Services." www.lesbiansandcancer.com/sup portandservices.htm.

Malecare. "Support Groups" (for men with breast cancer). www.malecare.com/ support_groups.htm.

Mautner Project, the National Lesbian Health Organization. "Support Group." www.mautnerproject.org.

Metastatic Breast Cancer Network. "Discussion Board." www.mbcnetwork.org/ page.aspx?nm=mainpage.

Mothers Supporting Daughters with Breast Cancer. "Get Support." www .mothersdaughters.org.

Out with Cancer. "LGBT Cancer Program Social Network." www.outwithcancer .com.

Schwarz, Roger. *The Skilled Facilitator*, 2nd ed. San Francisco, CA: Jossey-Bass, 2002.

SHARE. "Support Groups." www.sharecancersupport.org.

SHARE. "Ways We Can Help" (in English and Spanish). www.sharecancersup port.org/latina.php.

Sherman, Allen C., et al. "Patient Preferences Regarding Cancer Group Psycho-therapy Interventions: A View from the Inside." *Psychosomatics*, October 2007.

Sisters Network. Online support groups for African-American women. www.sis tersnetworkinc.org.

Weiss, Marisa, and Ellen Weiss. "Support Groups," in *Living Beyond Breast Cancer: A Survivor's Guide to When Treatment Ends and the Rest of Your Life Begins.* New York: Times Books, 1998.

Well Spouse Association. "Support Programs" (U.S. and Canadian sites for spousal caregivers). www.wellspouse.org/index.php?option=com_content&task=sect ion&id=8&Itemid=37.

Y-ME National Breast Cancer Organization. "Local Affiliates and Satellite Locations." www.y-me.org/affiliates/default.php.

Young Survival Coalition. "Programs" (for women under 40 with breast cancer). www.youngsurvival.org/programs/.

Chapter 16 — The 10 Best Questions for Financial Health After Breast Cancer

Asinof, Lynn. "Second Life: Survivors of Illnesses May Find Finances in Need of Care." *Wall Street Journal,* April 23, 1998.

Calder, Kimberly J., and Karen Pollitz. "What Cancer Survivors Need To Know About Health Insurance." www.canceradvocacy.org/resources/publications/insurance.pdf.

Cancerandcareers.org. *The Living and Working with Cancer Workbook,* 2nd ed. www.cancerandcareers.org/publications/.

Cancerandcareers.org. *The Most Important Resources for Working Women with Cancer.* www.cancerandcareers.org/publications/.

Cancerbackup. "Financial Issues." www.cancerbackup.org.uk/Resourcessupport/Practicalissues/Financiallegalissues/Financialissues.

CancerCare. *A Helping Hand,* 5th ed. (Resource guide). www.cancercare.org/get_help/assistance/helping_hand.php.

Citizen, The (U.K.), "Cancer Patients' Extra Worry," December 30, 2005.

CNNMoney.com. "Debt Reduction Planner." cgi.money.cnn.com/tools/debt planner/debtplanner.jsp.

DebtAdvice.org. "Consumer Advice." www.debtadvice.org.

Fayed, Lisa. "Financial Help for Cancer Patients: Where to Find Help for Cancer Care." cancer.about.com/od/treatmentoptions/a/cancerfinancial.htm.

Hoffman, Barbara. *Working It Out: Your Employment Rights as a Cancer Survivor.* National Coalition for Cancer Survivorship, 2003. www.canceradvocacy.org/resources/publications/employment.pdf.

Lankford, Kimberly. "Life Insurance for Cancer Survivors." www.kiplinger.com/columns/ask/archive/2006/q0803.htm.

Long, Marion. "How They Get By: What It's Like to Have Cancer Without Health Insurance." *MAMM Magazine,* March–April 2006. www.mamm.com.

Macmillan Cancer Support (U.K.). "Financial Help." www.macmillan.org.uk/Get_Support/Financial_help/Financial_help.aspx.

Mincer, Jilian. "Family Finances: Not So He~~~~

Wall S~~~~

~~~~upsi.org.

~~~~inancial Issues Related to Breast Cancer Care." cms.komen.org/Komen/AboutBreastCancer/Treatment/s_002802.

University of Florida Shands Cancer Center. "Financial and Insurance Issues." www.ufscc.ufl.edu/Patient/content.aspx?section=supportandresources&id= 18850.

USA Today, "Returning to Work After a Cancer Diagnosis," May 1, 2000.

U.S. Department of Health and Human Services, Centers for Medicare and Medicaid Services. Comprehensive information about Medicaid. www.cms.hhs. gov/home/medicaid.asp.

Weiman Hanks, Liza. *The Busy Family's Guide to Estate Planning: 10 Steps to Peace of Mind.* Berkeley, CA: Nolo Press, 2007.

Williams, Gurney, III, and Pamela Weintraub. "MAMM Special Report: The New Have-Nots: Are You One?" *MAMM Magazine*, January–February 2006. www .mamm.com.

Chapter 17—The 10 Best Questions
When Talking with Your Partner

Baker, Sherry. "Everything You Always Wanted to Know About Sex After Breast Cancer." *MAMM Magazine*, January–February 2006. www.mywire.com/ pubs/MAMM/2006/01/01/1179273/.

Balch, David. *Cancer for Two: A Caregiver's Perspective on Cancer.* Crest Park, CA: A Few Good People, 2006.

Breastcancer.org. "Sex and Intimacy: You and Your Partner." www.breastcancer .org/tips/intimacy/partner.jsp.

Brownworth, Victoria A. *Coming Out of Cancer: Writings from the Lesbian Cancer Epidemic.* New York: Seal Press, 2000.

Butler, Sandra, and Barbara Rosenblum. *Cancer in Two Voices*, 2nd ed. Midway, FL: Spinsters Ink Books, 1996.

Cancerbackup. "Effects of Hormonal Therapy on Sexuality." www.cancerbackup .org.uk/Resourcessupport/Relationshipscommunication/Sexuality/Hormonal therapy.

Cancerbackup. "How Chemotherapy Might Affect Your Sex Life." www.cancer backup.org.uk/Treatments/Chemotherapy/Sideeffects/Sexuality.

CancerCare. "Cancer, Intimacy and Relationship Concerns." www.cancercare.org/ reading_room/ask/archive/intimacy-archive.php.

Cole, Harriette, and John Pinderhughes. *Coming Together: Celebrations for African-American Families.* New York: Jump in the Sun Publishers, 2003.

Facing Breast Cancer Together. Support and research sites. fbctogether.org/fbc together/.

Kerr, Ian. *She Comes First: The Thinking Man's Guide to Pleasuring a Woman.* New York: Collins, 2004.

Kneece, Judy C. *Helping Your Mate Face Breast Cancer*, 6th ed. North Charleston, SC: Educare Publishing, 2007.

Kneece, Judy C. "Sexuality After Breast Cancer," in *Your Breast Cancer Treatment Handbook: Your Guide to Understanding the Disease, Treatment, Emotions, and Recovery from Breast Cancer*, 6th ed. North Charleston, SC: Educare Publishing, 2004.

Kydd, Sally, and Dana Rowett. *Intimacy after Cancer: A Woman's Guide.* Seattle: Big Think Media, 2006.

Lesbians and Breast Cancer Project Team for the Ontario Breast Cancer Community Research Initiative. *Coming Out About Lesbians and Cancer.* Ontario, 2004.

Long, Marion. "Dating After Breast Cancer." *MAMM Magazine.* March–April 2007. www.mamm.com.

Love, Susan, Karen Lindsey, and Marcia Williams. "Coping: Fears of Your Loved Ones," in *Dr. Susan Love's Breast Book,* 4th ed. Cambridge: Da Capo Press, 2005.

Memorial Sloan-Kettering Cancer Center. "A Guide for Caregivers." www.mskcc .org/mskcc/shared/graphics/survivorshipandsupport/Caregivers.pdf.

Memorial Sloan-Kettering Cancer Center. "Women, Cancer, and Sexual Health." www.mskcc.org/mskcc/html/56755.cfm.

Murcia, Andy, and Bob Stewart. *Man to Man.* New York: St. Martin's Press, 1989.

National Breast and Ovarian Cancer Centre (Australia). "Information for Partners." www.breasthealth.com.au/livingwithcancer/informationforpartners .html.

National Family Caregivers Association. "Tips and Guides for Caregivers." www .thefamilycaregiver.org/caregiving_resources/tips_and_guides.cfm.

Patient/Partner Project. "Free Resources for Patients and Partners." www.the patientpartnerproject.org.

Peck, Scott, and Shannon Peck. *The Love You Deserve: A Spiritual Guide to Genuine Love.* Solana Beach, CA: Lifepath Publishing, 2002.

Rayl, A. J. S. "Keeping It Together." *MAMM* ...

... ...er.pdf.

... ...ess. Intimacy, Sex and Your New Life," in *Living Beyond Breast Cancer: A Survivor's Guide to When Treatment Ends and the Rest of Your Life Begins.* New York: Times Books, 1998.

Well Spouse Foundation. Support for spousal caregivers. www.wellspouse.org.

Y-ME National Breast Cancer Organization. "When the Woman You Love Has Breast Cancer." www.y-me.org/publications/generalpubs/woman_you_love.php.

Chapter 18 — The 10 Best Questions
Before Breaking the News to Others

Breastcancer.org. "Dealing with Others' Unsettling Reactions." www.breastcancer.org/community/fears/ask_expert/2001_06/question_11.jsp.

Cancerandcareers.org. *Living and Working with Cancer Workbook,* 2nd ed. www.cancerandcareers.org/publications/.

Cancerandcareers.org. *The Most Important Resources for Working Women with Cancer.* www.cancerandcareers.org/publications/.

Kahn, Michael. "Gossip More Powerful than Truth Researchers Say," Yahoo News, October 15, 2007.

Keep Your Secrets. "Protect Your Privacy." www.keepyoursecrets.com.

Livestrong (Lance Armstrong Foundation). "Telling Others You Are a Survivor: Detailed Information." www.livestrong.org/site/c.khLXK1PxHmF/b.2660783/k.1951/Telling_Others_You_are_a_Survivor_Detailed_Information.htm.

Long, Marion, "Pretending to Be Fine." *MAMM Magazine,* July–August 2006. www.mamm.com.

Nash, Jennie. *The Victoria's Secret Catalog Never Stops Coming, and Other Lessons I Learned from Breast Cancer.* New York: Simon & Schuster, 2001.

Oken, Daniel. "What to Tell Cancer Patients: A Study of Medical Attitudes." *Journal of the American Medical Association.* 1961;175:1120–1128.

Ritchie, Karen. *Angels and Bolters: Women's Cancer Scripts.* Philadelphia: Xlibris, 2002.

Smith, Marty. "Words at Work." *The Advertiser*, February 11, 2005.

Wikicancer. "Telling People." www.wikicancer.org/page/Telling+people?t=anon.

Chapter 19 — The 10 Best Questions
Before Telling Your Children About Your Breast Cancer

Resources for Adults

American Cancer Society. "Helping Children When A Family Member Has Cancer: Dealing With A Parent's Terminal Illness." www.cancer.org/docroot/CRI/content/CRI_2_6x_Children_with_Cancer_in_the_Family_Dealing_with_a_Parents_Terminal_Illness.asp.

American Cancer Society. "Talking with Children About Cancer." www.cancer.org/docroot/ESN/content/ESN_2_1x_Talking_with_Children_About_Cancer.asp?sitearea=ESN.

Canadian Cancer Society. "Telling Children about a Cancer Diagnosis in the Family." www.cancer.ca/ccs/internet/standard/0,3182,3172_369293_990860910_langId-en,00.html.

Cancerbackup. "Talking to Children About Cancer." www.cancerbackup.org.uk/Resourcessupport/Relationshipscommunication/Talkingtochildren.

Carney, Karen L. *What Is Cancer Anyway? Explaining Cancer to Children of All Ages.* Wethersfield, CT: Dragonfly Publishing, 1998.

Fortin, Judy. "Honey, Mommy Has Cancer." www.cnn.com/2008/HEALTH/conditions/01/28/hm.cancer.kids/index.html.

Goldman, Linda. *Life and Loss: A Guide to Help Grieving Children,* 2nd ed. Philadelphia: Accelerated Development Publishers, 1999.

Love, Susan, Karen Lindsey, and Marcia Williams. "Coping: What to Tell Your Children," in *Dr. Susan Love's Breast Book,* 4th ed. Cambridge: Da Capo Press, 2005.

Russell, Michael. "Breast Cancer: Telling Your Kids About It." ezinearticles.com/?Breast-Cancer:-Telling-Your-Kids-About-It&id=376090.

Russell, Neil. *Can I Still Kiss You? Answering Your Children's Questions About Cancer.* Deerfield Beach, FL: Health Communications, 2001.

Van Dernoot, Peter, and Madelyn Case. *Helping Your Children Cope With Your Cancer: A Guide for Parents and Families,* 2nd. ed. Long Island City, NY: Hatherleigh Press, 2006.

Resources for Children

Children's Treehouse Foundation. Family support. www.childrenstreehousefdn.org.

Gellman, Marc, and Debbie Tilley. *Lost and Found: A Kid's Book for Living Through Loss.* New York: HarperCollins, 1999. Ages 9–12.

Kids Konnected. Support and education f...

...Cancer Organization. "Local Affiliates and Satellite Locations." www.y-me.org/affiliates/default.php.

Chapter 20 — The 10 Worst Questions to Ask a Breast Cancer Patient

Carr, Kris. "Cancer College," in *Crazy Sexy Cancer Tips*. Guilford, CT: Globe Pequot Press, 2007.

Clifford, Christine, and Jack Lindstrom. *Not Now, I'm Having a No Hair Day*. Minneapolis, MN: University of Minnesota Press, 1996.

Di Giacomo, Fran. *I'd Rather Do Chemo Than Clean Out the Garage: Choosing Laughter over Tears*. Dallas: Brown Books, 2003.

Elsagher, Brenda. *If the Battle Is Over, Why Am I Still in Uniform?* Andover, MN: Expert Publishing, 2003.

Gelman, Patty, and Leslie Zemsky. *Humor After the Tumor: One Woman's Look at Her Year with Breast Cancer*. Amherst, NY: Prometheus Books, 2003.

Humor Project, The. *The 2008 Sourcebook from the Humor Project, Inc.* www.humor project.com/publications/sourcebook.pdf.

Jest for the Health of It! Humor resources. www.jesthealth.com.

Klein, Allen. *The Courage to Laugh*. New York: Tarcher/Putnam Books, 1998.

Klein, Allen. *The Healing Power of Humor*. New York: Tarcher/Putnam Books, 1989.

Learning Place Online.com. "Are You Ready for Cancer Jokes?" www.learning placeonline.com/illness/humor/jokes-intro.htm.

Sherman, James R. *The Magic of Humor in Caregiving*. Golden Valley, MN: Pathway Books, 1995.

University of Michigan Comprehensive Cancer Center. "Humor and Cancer." www.cancer.med.umich.edu/support/humor_and_cancer.shtml.

Walker Jensen, Laura. *Thanks for the Mammogram! Fighting Cancer with Faith, Hope and a Healthy Dose of Laughter*. Grand Rapids, MI: Revell, 2006.

Wooten, Patty. *Compassionate Laughter: Jest for Your Health*, 2nd ed. Santa Cruz, CA: JestHealth, 2000.

Jennifer L. A. Armstrong, M.D., is a breast cancer medical oncologist with Paoli Hematology Oncology Associates in Paoli, Pennsylvania. She is a member of Breastcancer.org's Physician Advisory Board and on the board of directors for Living Beyond Breast Cancer (LBBC). Dr. Armstrong has a special interest in physicians' communication skills.

J. B. Askew, M.D., is a board-certified pathologist in private practice at the Houston Northwest Medical Center in Houston, Texas. He has more than 35 years of experience as a pathologist and wrote a popular article to help breast cancer patients understand their pathology reports. His article is available at www .breastpath.com/pathrep.htm.

Dave Balch of Twin Peaks, California, is on a mission to help the partners of cancer patients cope with caring for their loved ones and themselves as caregivers. His award-winning work is based on his experiences in helping his wife, Chris, battle cancer. He has authored the book *Cancer for Two: An Inspiring True Story and Guide for Cancer Patients and Their Partners*, and founded a cancer support organization called the Patient/Partner Project. His Web site is www .thepatientpartnerproject.org.

Stephen Barrett, M.D., a retired psychiatrist in Allentown, Pennsylvania, is an author, editor, and consumer advocate best known for his popular and informative Web site, Quackwatch. Quackwatch, Inc., is a nonprofit organization whose mission is to "combat health-related frauds, myths, fads, fallacies, and misconduct" while providing "quackery-related information that is difficult or impossible to get elsewhere." His Web site is www.quackwatch.org.

Robert C. Bast, Jr., M.D., is the vice president for Translational Research at the M. D. Anderson Cancer Center, University of Texas in Houston. He cares for breast and ovarian cancer patients and specializes in helping new cancer treatments move from the laboratory to the clinic. Dr. Bast has been listed in the *Best Doctors of America* and in *America's Top Physicians*. The Web site is www .mdanderson.org.

Hamilton Beazley, Ph.D., is Scholar-in-Residence at St. Edward's University in Austin, Texas, and author of *No Regrets: A Ten-Step Program for Living in the*

Present and Leaving the Past Behind. Dr. Beazley has been interviewed on *Oprah*, NBC, CNN, and many other television and radio shows. The Web site is www.stedwards.edu.

Norman Berk is a Certified Financial Planner and the founder of Professional Asset Strategies, Inc., in Birmingham, Alabama. Both he and his wife are cancer survivors. Mr. Berk founded a charitable organization called The Breast Cancer Research Foundation and is on the Professional Advisory Board for breastcancer.org. His Web site is http://proassetsllc.com.

Lorraine Biros, L.C.P.C. is a Licensed Clinical Professional Counselor and the director for Client Services at the Mautner Project: The National Lesbian Health Organization in Washington, D.C. The Mautner Project provides support for lesbians with cancer and their partners and caregivers. Ms. Biros has more than 28 years of counseling experience in the lesbian and gay community. The Web site of the Mautner Project is www.mautnerproject.org.

Peter Block has an international reputation as a management consultant and is the author of best-selling books, including *Flawless Consulting: A Guide to Getting Your Expertise Used*, and *The Answer to How Is Yes*, a book that examines underlying assumptions about asking questions. His newest book is *Community: The Structure of Belonging*, and his Web site is www.peterblock.com.

Albert L. Blumberg, M.D., is a board-certified radiation oncologist and Vice Chair of the Department of Radiation Oncology at the Greater Baltimore Medical Center in Baltimore, Maryland. He has been practicing all aspects of adult radiation oncology for more than 30 years. The Web site is www.gbmc .org.

Winfield (Win) A. Boerckel, L.C.S.W.-R., M.S.W., M.B.A., is a licensed clinical oncology social worker in New York who has counseled hundreds of cancer patients and their families for more than 12 years at CancerCare, a top cancer support and education source. He is also CancerCare's LiveStrong National Relations Program Director. The Web site for CancerCare is www.cancercare .org.

Deborah Bruner, Ph.D., R.N., has more than 17 years of experience with major clinical trials sponsored by the National Cancer Institute, and is the director at the Abramson Cancer Center of the University of Pennsylvania, a leading organization in cancer care and research located in Philadelphia. Dr. Bruner is also a professor of nursing. The Web site is www.upenn.edu.

Joanna Bull, M.A., M.F.C.C., was Gilda Radner's psychotherapist during the comedian's battle with cancer. A pioneer in the concept of cancer support communities, Ms. Bull is the co-founder (along with Gene Wilder and the late Joel Siegel) of Gilda's Club Worldwide, with a network across North America of meeting places, support groups, and special educational programs for men women child . . .

. . . director of *Ebony*

magazine. She is also the president and creative director of Harriette Cole Productions, and coaches recording artists, including notable musicians such as JoJo, Alicia Keys, and Mary J. Blige. Her Web site is www.harriettecole.com and her Wikipedia entry is at http://en.wikipedia.org/wiki/Harriette_Cole.

Karen Collins, M.S., R.D., C.D.N., is a registered dietician and nutrition advisor to the American Institute for Cancer Research, an organizational pioneer in researching cancer-related diet and nutrition located in Washington, D.C. The Web site for the institute is www.aicr.org.

Melissa Craft, Ph.D., R.N., is an Advanced Oncology Certified Nurse at Breast Imaging of Oklahoma in Edmond, Oklahoma. Dr. Craft has more than 27 years experience in specialized nursing care for cancer patients and is a professor of nursing at the University of Oklahoma. The Web site is www.breastimagingofoklahoma.com.

Gregory O. Dick, M.D., F.A.C.S., is a board-certified plastic surgeon in Rockville, Maryland. Dr. Dick is a former president of the Maryland chapter of the American Cancer Society and a past chief of surgery at Shady Grove Hospital in Rockville. His Web site is www.gregorydickmd.com.

Brenda Elsagher is a cancer survivor in Burnsville, Minnesota, who has turned her medical experiences into a new career as a stand-up comedian and cancer humor author. Her inspirational story is featured on the National Cancer Institute's Web site. Ms. Elsagher is the author of several books, including *If the Battle Is Over, Why Am I Still in Uniform?* Her Web site is www.livingand laughing.com.

Betty Ferrell, Ph.D., is a nurse and researcher at the City of Hope National Medical Center in Los Angeles, California, a leading cancer care and research center. Dr. Ferrell has more than 30 years experience as an oncology nurse and her research focuses on quality-of-life issues. She has the unusual distinction of holding graduate degrees in both nursing and theology. The Web site is www .cityofhope.org.

Patricia Ganz, M.D., is the Director of Cancer Prevention and Control Research at UCLA's Jonsson Comprehensive Cancer Center in Los Angeles, a professor, and a member of the Institute of Medicine. Dr. Ganz has devoted the past 25 years to the study of quality-of-life outcomes in cancer, including research on the emotional impact of breast cancer. The Web site is www.cancer.ucla.edu.

John Gray, Ph.D., is the world's number-one-selling relationship author. An international gender and relationship expert, his *New York Times* best-selling book series *Men Are from Mars, Women Are from Venus* has sold over 30 million copies worldwide. Gray's internationally acclaimed Mars-Venus principles have helped millions of couples to understand the differences between men and women. Dr. Gray's latest book is available at www.marsvenus.com/collide and his Wikipedia entry is at http://en.wikipedia.org/wiki/John_Gray_(U.S._author).

Julie R. Heiman, Ph.D., is the Director of the famous Kinsey Institute for Research in Sex, Gender and Reproduction at Indiana University in Bloomington, Indiana. For more than 60 years, the Kinsey Institute has been the worldwide pioneer and leader in human sexuality, gender, and reproduction research. Dr. Heiman's research interests include sexual arousal and traumatic sexual experiences. The Web site of the Kinsey Institute is www.kinseyinstitute.org.

Bruce J. Hillman, M.D., is a professor of radiology at the University of Virginia's School of Medicine in Charlottesville. A medical imaging specialist and radiology researcher, Dr. Hillman is on the National Cancer Institute's Advisory Board for Clinical Trials. The Web site is www.virginia.edu.

Clifford A. Hudis, M.D., is the chief of the Breast Cancer Medicine Service at Memorial Sloan-Kettering Cancer Center in New York City. He is also a professor in the Department of Medicine at Cornell Medical College. His research interests include chemotherapy, hormone therapy, and other systemic treatment modalities. The Web site is www.mskcc.org.

Alex Keller, M.D., is a board-certified plastic surgeon in New York City with more than 25 years experience. Dr. Keller specializes in DIEP flap surgeries for breast reconstruction following mastectomies. His Web site is www.breastflap.com.

Beverly Kirkhart is co-author of *Chicken Soup for the Surviving Soul: 101 Healing Stories About Those Who Have Survived Cancer*, and a breast cancer survivor since 1993. Ms. Kirkhart lives in Santa Barbara, California, authored *My Healing Companion*, and is a frequent motivational keynote speaker. Her Web site is www.beverlykirkhart.com.

Richard Koonce is president of Richard Koonce Productions, a human resources consulting and communications firm in Brookline, Massachusetts. Mr. Koonce is an experienced writer, consultant, facilitator, coach, and interviewer and has ~~author~~...

...~~graphy is at http://~~ en.wikipedia.org/wiki/C._Everett_Koop.

Sally Kydd, Psy.D., L. Psych., is a clinical psychologist and a breast cancer survivor based in Hong Kong and New Jersey. Dr. Kydd believes that a woman's sexuality after a diagnosis of cancer is frequently misunderstood and underappreciated. She is the co-author of the book *Intimacy after Cancer: A Woman's Guide*. Her Web site is http://intimacyaftercancer.com.

Claudia Lee is the principal of C. Z. Lee and Associates in Hudson, New York, and is a member of Breastcare.org's Advisory Council and other national organizations. Ms. Lee specializes in consultations with institutions planning comprehensive breast programs.

Susan Love, M.D., is a "breast guru," surgeon, teacher, and Medical Director of a nonprofit organization, Dr. Susan Love Research Foundation, dedicated to eradicating cancer. Dr. Love is the author of the bestseller, *Dr. Susan Love's Breast Book*, 4th ed. She counsels breast cancer patients on all aspects of their disease. Dr. Love's Web site is www.drsusanloveresearchfoundation.org.

Cicily Carson Maton is a Certified Financial Planner™ and the founder of Aequus Wealth Management Resources, a Chicago-based financial planning and investment firm that specializes in advising people in major life transitions. She has appeared several times on the television show *Right on the Money*. Her Web site is www.aequuswealth.com.

Musa Mayer is a breast cancer survivor, patient advocate, and author of three books on breast cancer. She publishes frequently in medical journals and consumer magazines, works with the FDA and the Institute of Medicine, and runs two Web sites devoted to supporting women with advanced breast cancer, www.advancedbc.org and www.brainmetsbc.org.

Rear Admiral Kenneth P. Moritsugu, M.D., M.P.H., retired as Acting U.S. Surgeon General in 2007. Admiral Moritsugu's 40-year career in public health includes many honors and his service as an Assistant Surgeon General beginning with Surgeon General C. Everett Koop in 1988, and as Deputy Surgeon General for nearly 10 years. Admiral Moritsugu's Wikipedia biography is at http://en.wikipedia.org/wiki/Kenneth_P._Moritsugu. The U.S. Surgeon General's Web site is www.surgeongeneral.gov.

Jennie Nash is a breast cancer survivor and writer living near Los Angeles, California. She has authored several books, including, *The Victoria's Secret Catalog Never Stops Coming, and Other Lessons I Learned From Breast Cancer*, where she describes how breast cancer made her "a wise old woman at the age of 36," and a novel featuring a breast cancer survivor, *The Last Beach Bungalow.* Her Web site is www.jennienash.com.

Debbie Nigro is an award-winning radio personality, champion of women, author, speaker, and business executive based in New York. Ms. Nigro has interviewed hundreds of people for her radio shows, which are aired in 450 markets. She is also a consultant to the producers of the Broadway show, *The First Wives Club Musical.* Ms. Nigro's video, posts, and blogs are at www.firstwivesworld.com.

Anna Nowak, M.D., is a medical oncologist and researcher at Sir Charles Gairdner Hospital in Perth, Western Australia. She has been an oncologist for more than 11 years, participates in guideline development for Australia's National Breast Cancer Center, and has been awarded major research grants. The Web site is www.scgh.health.wa.gov.au.

Dr. Scott Peck and Shannon Peck of Solana Beach, California, are the co-founders of TheLoveCenter.com, an educational organization dedicated to raising relationship and spiritual awareness, co-hosts of a national radio show, *Love Talk*, and co-authors of several love and relationship books, including *The Love You Deserve: A Spiritual Guide to Genuine Love.* Their Web site is www.thelovecenter.com.

Edith A. Perez, M.D., is the director of the Clinical Cancer Research Study Unit and Breast Cancer Program at the Mayo Clinic in Jacksonville, Florida. She received her medical degree from the University of Puerto Rico. Dr. Perez is widely published in her research areas, including gene therapy and hormone therapies for breast cancer. The Web site is www.mayoclinic.org.

Vicki Rackner, M.D., is a board-certified surgeon who left the operating room to help patients, patients' families, and caregivers partner more effectively with their doctors through her company, Medical Bridges. She is also an author, speaker, and consultant, including co-authoring a *Chicken Soup for the Soul: Healthy Living Series* book and several patient self-help books. Her Web site is www.MedicalBridges.com.

Betty Rollin is a former NBC correspondent, award-winning journalist, and the author of *Last Wish* and *First, You Cry*, a groundbreaking book and cancer classic that she wrote in 1976 to tell about her breast cancer and mastectomy. Ms. Rollin is also a co-author of *Here's the Bright Side: Of Failure, Fear, Cancer, Di-*

...... patient care for more than 22 years. The Web site is www.jointcommission.org.

Susan Sikora hosts a locally produced TV talk show in San Francisco, California, called "Bay Area Focus with Susan Sikora" and has interviewed hundreds of political, entertainment, and health celebrities on her show. Ms. Sikora is an Emmy winner who has formerly hosted live TV talk shows for PBS, CBS, NBC, and ABC. The Web site is http://cwbayarea.com.

Pat Spicer, L.C.S.W., a licensed social worker in New York, has specialized in helping cancer patients cope with their emotional, personal, relationship, and medical issues for more than 20 years. She is currently at CancerCare, a top cancer support organization and was formerly a social worker at Memorial Sloan-Kettering Cancer Center. The Web site is www.cancercare.org.

Susan Stamberg is an internationally-known broadcast journalist and an award-winning special correspondent for National Public Radio. She has been inducted into the Broadcasting Hall of Fame and the Radio Hall of Fame and is a breast cancer survivor. The Web site is www.npr.org. Ms. Stamburg's Wikipedia biography is at http://en.wikipedia.org/wiki/Susan_Stamberg.

Helen Thomas is a legendary question asker, a news service reporter, Hearst Newspapers columnist, and member of the White House Press Corps. She has served for 57 years as a correspondent and White House bureau chief for United Press International (UPI). Ms. Thomas has covered every president since John F. Kennedy and is famous for challenging presidents from her front row seat during press conferences. Ms. Thomas's Wikipedia biography is at http://en.wikipedia.org/wiki/Helen_Thomas.

Todd Tuttle, M.D., is the Chief of Surgical Oncology at the University of Minnesota in the Twin Cities area. His publications include a 2007 study of double mastectomies. Dr. Tuttle is a graduate of the Johns Hopkins School of Medicine and completed his fellowship in surgical oncology at the M.D. Anderson Cancer Center in Texas. The Web site is www.umn.edu.

Edward O. Uthman, M.D., is a practicing pathologist at the OakBend Medical Center, a community hospital in Richmond, Texas. With over 30 years experience as a doctor, Dr. Uthman is also an adjunct professor at the University of

Texas's School of Medicine. His online article, *CancerGuide: The Biopsy Report: A Patient's Guide* is available at http://cancerguide.org/pathology.html.

Marisa C. Weiss, M.D., is the president and founder of the nonprofit organization breastcancer.org, which provides the world's leading online resource for breast health and breast cancer at www.breastcancer.org. She is the co-author with her mother of *Living Beyond Breast Cancer*, the author of *7 Minutes! How to Get the Most from Your Doctor Visit*, and co-author with her teenage daughter of the new book *Taking Care of Your "Girls": A Breast Health Guide for Girls, Teens, and In-Betweens*. Dr. Weiss is also the director of Breast Radiation Oncology and of Breast Health Outreach at Lankenau Hospital in the Philadelphia area.

Shawna C. Willey, M.D., is a breast surgeon and the director of the Betty Lou Ourisman Breast Health Center, Department of Surgery at the Georgetown University Hospital in Washington, D.C. Dr. Willey has devoted the last nine years to specializing in breast surgery and is the 2008 President of the American Society of Breast Surgeons. The Web site is www.georgetown.edu.